FAT

In contemporary western societies the fat body has become a focus of stigmatizing discourses and practices aimed at disciplining, regulating and containing it. Despite the fact that in many western countries fat bodies outnumber those that are thin, fat people are still socially marginalized and treated with derision and even repulsion. Medical and public health experts insist that an 'obesity epidemic' exists and that fatness is a pathological condition which should be prevented and controlled.

Fat is a book about why the fat body has become so reviled and viewed as diseased, the target of such intense discussion and debate about ways to reduce its size down to socially and medically acceptable dimensions. It is also about the lived experience of fat embodiment: how does it feel to be fat in a fat-phobic society? Deborah Lupton explores fat as a cultural artefact: a bodily substance or body shape that is given meaning by complex and shifting systems of ideas, practices, emotions, material objects and interpersonal relationships.

Fat reviews current scholarship and research into obesity discourse and politics, drawing upon critical perspectives offered in the humanities and social sciences and by fat activism and the size acceptance movement. It will be an engaging introduction for the interested general reader, as well as for students across the humanities and social sciences.

Deborah Lupton is in the Department of Sociology and Social Policy, University of Sydney. She is an internationally renowned sociologist and the author/co-author of eleven other books, including *Medicine as Culture, Risk, Risk and Everyday Life* (with J. Tulloch), *The Imperative of Health, The New Public Health* (with A. Petersen) and *Food, the Body and the Self*. Her curre   ultural dimensions of medicine,   he family.

SHORTCUTS – *'Little Books on Big Issues'*

Shortcuts is a major new series of concise, accessible introductions to some of the major issues of our times. The series is developed as an A to Z coverage of emergent or new social, cultural and political phenomenon. Issues and topics covered range from food to fat, from climate change to suicide bombing, from love to zombies. Whilst the principal focus of *Shortcuts* is the relevance of current issues, topics and debates to the social sciences and humanities, the books should also appeal to a wider audience seeking guidance on how to engage with today's leading social, political and philosophical debates.

Series Editor: Anthony Elliott is Director of the Hawke Research Institute, where he is Research Professor of Sociology at the University of South Australia.

Titles in the series:

Confronting Climate Change
Constance Lever-Tracy

Feelings
Stephen Frosh

Suicide Bombings
Riaz Hassan

Web 2.0
Sam Han

Global Finance
Robert J. Holton

Freedom
Nick Stevenson

Planet Sport
Kath Woodward

Fat
Deborah Lupton

Reinvention
Anthony Elliott

Panic
Keith Tester

FAT

Deborah Lupton

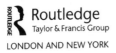

Routledge
Taylor & Francis Group

LONDON AND NEW YORK

First published 2013
by Routledge
2 Park Square, Milton Park, Abingdon, Oxon OX14 4RN

Simultaneously published in the USA and Canada
by Routledge
711 Third Avenue, New York, NY 10017

*Routledge is an imprint of the Taylor & Francis Group,
an informa business*

British Library Cataloguing in Publication Data
A catalogue record for this book is available from the
British Library

Library of Congress Cataloging-in-Publication Data
Lupton, Deborah
Fat / Deborah Lupton
p. cm. – (Short cuts)
Includes bibliographical references and index.
1. Obesity. 2. Obesity–Epidemiology. 3. Obesity–Social
aspects. I. Title
RA645.O23L85 2013
614.5'9398–dc23   2012011337

ISBN: 978-0-415-52443-8 (hbk)
ISBN: 978-0-415-52444-5 (pbk)
ISBN: 978-0-203-10065-3 (ebk)

Typeset in Bembo
by Taylor & Francis Books

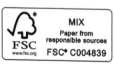

Printed and bound in Great Britain by the MPG Books Group

CONTENTS

SHORTCUTS – *'Little Books on Big Issues'*

Series editor's preface

Shortcuts is a major new series of concise, accessible introductions to some of the major issues of our times. The series is developed as an A to Z coverage of emergent or new social, cultural and political phenomenon. Issues and topics covered range from food to fat, from climate change to suicide bombing, from love to zombies. Whilst the principal focus of **Shortcuts** is the relevance of current issues, topics and debates to the social sciences and humanities, the books should also appeal to a wider audience seeking guidance on how to engage with today's leading social, political and philosophical debates.

Ours is a culture of the fat-phobic. In a 24/7 world of mass media, shaped to its core by consumerism, corporatism and celebrity culture, there an endless dissection and scrutiny of fat (and the possible emergence of fat) bodies. As Deborah Lupton charts in this book with sociological flair, the categorizing of people as fat represents a perverse cultural blend of terror and delight. In Fat, Lupton examines the complex interconnections between bodies, food and obesity, as well as society's triumphant casting of fat as worthy of contempt, horror and commercial exploitation. From daily media scrutiny of celebrity bodies for any signs of weight gain to women and men's anxieties that their diets are making them fat, Lupton's analysis is written with remarkable clarity and insight. This book offers a vital shortcut on an issue of pressing public political significance.

Anthony Elliott

1
INTRODUCTION

One night, while channel-surfing, I came across an episode of the American version of *The Biggest Loser* reality television series. It seemed to be the final for that series, as three contestants were presented as competing to be the ultimate winner. I watched in horrified fascination for a time as the 'journey' of each of these three was detailed in flashback accounts. The focus on humiliating, vilifying and punishing the contestants in the programme was overwhelming. It was shown how the contestants at the beginning of the series, and for each week during it, displayed their bodies dressed only in skimpy, stretchy bra-tops and shorts for women and brief shorts for men. This apparel allowed their rolls of wobbly flesh to be fully on display to the studio and television audience. One flashback showed each contestant's initial experience of a public weigh-in in the first episode of the series. They stepped onto scales and their extreme weight was displayed in giant letters, establishing the gargantuan nature of the task that lay ahead – to lose enough weight to be considered 'normal'.

The contestants' mortification and humiliation at their fat bodies being displayed was obvious by the expression on their faces and the words they spoke. At the moment of first exposure of her obesity, for example, one woman exclaimed how 'disgusted' she was at her own body. The flashbacks showed how the contestants' flesh was punished each day by cruel exercise routines, with thin and taut-bodied personal trainers shouting with hostility at them to 'encourage' them to work their bodies harder. The contestants were shown sweating, beetroot-faced, and, in one case, vomiting from the exertion, loudly exclaiming about the pain and suffering they were undergoing. Nonetheless, in the final episode all three finalists declared that 'it was worth the pain'. They had each lost a huge amount of weight and looked, if not thin, then at least 'average' sized. They commented that by shedding their weight, they 'had their lives back', as if their fat bodies had previously controlled their destinies.

The 2012 season of the Australian *The Biggest Loser* focused on the loneliness and despair endured by the contestants, who were particularly selected because they lacked a life partner and allegedly were desperately 'looking for love'. Not only were they forced to expose their semi-naked bodies to the viewing audience as part of the ritual weigh-in process, they were also encouraged to bare their souls. Thus, for example, an advance television promotion for the series showed one of the male contestants sitting on a stool gesturing to his body and saying 'Look at me – no-one loves this!' Another male contestant was shown commenting that 'I'm ready for love' as the words 'Love yourself' scrolled across the screen.

The underlying meanings of this programme are all too clear. Fat people are lonely, unloved, emotionally volatile and sad; they deserve punishing exercise routines and stringent diets as part of their weight-loss efforts; they are childish and need a stern authority figure to force them into proper weight-loss habits. The focus on love in the 2012 Australian *The Biggest Loser* season combined two ideas: that fat people do not love themselves, or else they would not have allowed themselves to become fat, and that no-one else is sexually attracted to them because of their fat bodies. Such people are represented as objects of both pity and contempt.

As these and other public displays of humiliation of fat people suggest, in contemporary western societies the fat body has become a focus of stigmatizing discourses and practices aimed at disciplining, normalizing and containing it. Despite the fact that in many western countries fat bodies outnumber those that are thin, fat people are still socially marginalized and treated with derision and even repulsion. It seems that there is something culturally repellent about the fat body, something that calls out to be controlled, contained and punished. In popular and expert representations, fat people are portrayed as having 'let themselves go' not only literally but also symbolically. Their bodies are viewed as grotesque, uncontained, physical evidence of their inability to control their desires and greed. Their flesh bulges, burgeons forth, takes up more space than other bodies, provoking negative attention in its excessiveness. Their fatness overwhelms their identity, to the point that others see only the fat and not the 'real person inside', as one of the American *The Biggest Loser* contestants put it.

Fat is a book about why the fat body is so reviled, the target of such intense discussion and debate about ways to reduce its size down to socially and medically acceptable dimensions. It is also about the lived experience of fat embodiment: how it feels to be fat in a fat-phobic society. Above all, this book is about fat as a cultural artefact: a bodily substance or body shape that in the particular context of late modern western societies in the early decades of the twenty-first century is given meaning by complex and shifting systems of discourses, practices, emotions, material objects and interpersonal relationships. In and of itself, fat has no meaning. It is the specific historical, social and cultural context in which fatness is lived, experienced, portrayed and regulated which give it meaning, just as other bodily attributes or features such as skin or hair colour, youth and height take on certain meanings depending on their context. These meanings are dynamic and shifting, subject to change as the context changes.

The emergence of the 'obesity epidemic'

Fatness has been the subject of intense interest since the final decade of the twentieth century. Beginning from that time, medical and public health experts and researchers began to publish extensively about what has become commonly referred to as the 'obesity epidemic' or the 'obesity crisis'. While the fat body has long been associated with ill-health in medicine and public health, this period witnessed an unprecedented intensification of focus by these experts and researchers on the negative health and economic effects of obesity. The mid 2000s appear to be a pivotal point at which intense concern about the 'obesity epidemic' intensified and peaked. *Time* magazine named 2004 'The Year of Obesity'. That year the World Health Organization's *Global Strategy on Diet, Physical Activity and Health* was released and the Centers for Disease Control predicted that a poor diet and lack of exercise would soon claim more lives than tobacco-related disease in the United States (Herrick 2009: 53).

Medical and public health reports since the 1990s have asserted that far more people are now overweight or obese compared with past eras, that this is associated with a greater incidence of illness, disease and premature mortality and therefore a greater burden has been placed upon the health care system of those countries seen to be affected, which include most of the developed world. Some public health experts have also contended that a global obesity pandemic is emerging in which the dietary habits of western nations are beginning to be taken up in developing countries, causing increasing numbers of people in those countries to gain excess weight. These pronouncements drew the attention of the news media, which seized upon this apparent new health crisis as eminently newsworthy and have produced a multitude of news reports on the topic. Governments have sponsored forums, developed taskforces, strategic plans and commissions and produced policy documents directed at dealing with the obesity crisis; health promotion programmes have been funded to inform people about the problem and what to do about it; and weight-control interventions designed for schools and workplaces have been developed and implemented. The commercial sector, for its part, has taken the opportunity to develop and market products aimed at weight loss for populations who were becoming increasingly aware of the obesity-related health risks publicized in the above forums.

Critical weight studies/fat studies

In response to the emergence of obesity as an apparent new and urgent health crisis, a significant number of researchers and writers within the social sciences and humanities have developed a strong interest in fatness from a critical and analytical perspective. While critical explorations of the ways in which fat people are represented and treated in expert and popular cultures have been published since the late 1960s, particularly by fat activist groups, it is only relatively recently, in tandem with the increasing medicalization and pathologizing of fatness, that a significant body of literature has begun to emerge and gain coherence as a field of study. Since the turn of this century several conferences have been devoted to the critical analysis of obesity discourse. A number of interesting book-length works, both monographs and edited collections, have been published addressing the social, cultural, historical and political aspects of fatness, as well as a large and ever-growing number of scholarly journal articles.

Before going any further it is important to discuss here the terminology around the choice made to use the terms 'fat', 'overweight' or 'obese'. This choice has become increasingly political and contentious in the context of the emergence of fat activism. Many academics and activists prefer the term 'fat' to 'overweight' or 'obese', which 'O-words' (Wann 2009: xii) they associate with normative and pathologizing connotations. They see 'obesity' in particular as an officious medical term which designates fatness as pathology by its very use. Thus, to describe someone as 'obese' immediately places that person within the purview of medicine as someone who has the disease of 'obesity' and is therefore considered abnormal, inevitably unhealthy or at high risk of disease and thus as requiring medical intervention to reduce his or her weight. Fat activists also reject the terms 'underweight', 'normal weight' and 'overweight' because they suggest that there is an ideal, non-deviant weight to which people should aspire (Rothblum 2012). Just as gays, lesbians, bisexual and transgendered people chose to reappropriate the once pejorative word 'queer' for their own purposes, attempting to reinstate it as a positive self-identifying and political term, some academics and activists seek to use the word 'fat' to describe corpulent people in a positive, accepting manner. Such writers, although acknowledging the pejorative connotations of 'fat' which have developed over centuries of stigmatizing and moralistic portrayals of the fat body, view the term as at least outside the medical sphere of influence. As Marilyn Wann (2009: xii), a well-known American fat activist, claims, '[t]here is nothing negative or rude in the word fat unless someone makes the effort to put it there; using the word fat as a descriptor (not a discriminator) can help dispel prejudice.' In an acknowledgement of the political nature of the terminology around body weight, in this book I have also chosen to use the term 'fat' rather than 'obese' or 'overweight'.

Such is the growing popularity of adopting the word 'fat' to describe corpulent embodiment that a specific field of research-ing and teaching in academia entitled 'fat studies' has emerged. It now has its own academic journal, *Fat Studies*, first published in 2012, a sign from the publishers and editorial board at least of the belief that there will be scholarly interest in this area for some time to come. Alternatively, some scholars writing in this area prefer to describe their work with the rubric of 'critical weight studies' or 'critical obesity studies'. The emphasis in these terms is on the word 'critical', as these scholars seek to identify and challenge the taken-for-granted assumptions circulating in mainstream lay discourses and in the biomedical and public health literature on obesity/fatness.

Constructing 'obesity'

One of the major contentions of critical writers on fatness concerns the socially constructed nature of the 'obesity epidemic': hence the common use in this literature of scare quotes around this phrase to denote its contested meaning. As scholars in the humanities and social sciences have argued for many years, biomedical and public health knowledges are not transparent, comprised of pre-existing 'truths' which simply wait to be 'discovered' by researchers. Rather, as is the case for any kind of knowledge, these knowledge systems are socially and culturally constructed, given meaning through researchers' decisions about which topics are important to research, the methods they use to collect data and the ways in which these data are analysed and interpreted. From this perspective, all diseases, illnesses and physical conditions are also social constructions. By this I do not mean that they do not have biological, fleshly manifestations. It is rather to contend that these physical manifestations inevitably are interpreted and thus experienced in certain ways based on pre-existing assumptions and belief systems which themselves are open to constant change.

This approach to medical knowledge, illness and disease has itself been influenced by a robust literature addressing the sociology and anthropology of the body which has developed over the past three decades. Writers focusing on the sociology and anthropology of the body are interested in exploring the ways in which the human body is a complex admixture of biology, society and culture. They have been influenced by poststructuralist perspectives on the relationship between social processes, discourse and power relations, and particularly the insights offered in the work of the French philosopher-historian Michel Foucault. The concept of 'discourse' in poststructuralist thought is understood broadly as defined and coherent ways of representing and discussing people, events or things, as expressed in a range of forums, from everyday talk to the popular media and the internet to expert talk and texts. Discourses are contextual, embedded in particular historical, political and cultural settings. Discourses both reflect common understandings and perpetuate them, contributing to ways of thinking about, living and treating our bodies.

The concept of discourse is frequently employed as a conceptual term in fat studies/critical weight studies. Such analyses are not simply about deconstructing the discursive dimensions of fatness; they also seek to identify the power dimensions involved in such representations. Questions such as the following are often asked by those engaging in fat studies/critical weight studies: whose interests are served by the reproduction of dominant discourses on fatness? How is the distinction between Self and Other maintained by these discourses? How might these discourses be resisted or subverted?

A poststructuralist perspective on fatness contends that the condition of 'obesity' did not exist before a decision was made that a certain constellation of bodily characteristics should be given this label. The very label of 'obesity' as it is bestowed upon individuals depends on the construction of the Body Mass Index (BMI) measurement, which is the result of a decision made to use specific bodily characteristics in a defined mathematical formula to produce a number. Decisions again were made to select arbitrary 'cut-off' points to denote 'underweight', 'normal weight', 'overweight' and 'obesity'. When these cut-off points were lowered, again due to an arbitrary decision, many more people became designated as 'obese' and therefore categorized as diseased and susceptible to manifold health risks, even though their body mass remained the same as before this change. Likewise, the 'obesity epidemic' did not exist before certain ways of collecting and interpreting data across the population were brought into play. Such decisions are always social, cultural, historical and very often political.

Critical scholarship on obesity and fatness also draws upon the sociological literature on medicalization by identifying and criticizing the tendency of medicine to bring certain bodily phenomena or social problems under its aegis, thus rendering them susceptible to medical definitions and treatment. History is replete with examples of conditions that once were considered 'medical problems' or 'diseases' by the medical profession but which then lost their medicalized status. The emergence of fatness as a 'medical problem' shares features with other conditions that once were medicalized and pathologized, such as hysteria or homosexuality.

Anthropologists use the term 'culture-bound syndrome' to describe the sociocultural construction of disease categories. A disease or condition is considered 'culture-bound' if it is specific to a belief system operating in a particular cultural context: a certain country, for example, or subgroup within a geographical area. It has been contended by some anthropologists that obesity is such a culture-bound syndrome, specific to the contemporary western cultural context. They have pointed out that the condition of 'obesity' is reliant both upon the beliefs that fatness is unhealthy and a physical manifestation of weak will and lack of self-discipline and upon the requisite technologies (scales, measuring tapes, dietary guidelines and so on) to measure, define and treat it (Ritenbaugh 1982). Anthropologists have also observed that in contrast to contemporary western society, in several non-western cultures fatness is viewed as a physically desirable attribute, a sign of good health and wellbeing and certainly not a marker of illness or deviance (Kulick and Meneley 2005). Indeed historians have made similar observations of concepts of fatness in western societies in past eras (Gilman 2010).

Fatness itself is a dynamic and shifting state in lay views and in medical culture. While, for example, the BMI is used clinically to label people as 'overweight' or 'obese', and thus is very precise in identifying people who fit these categories, notions of fatness are multiple, contingent and relative. Thus, for example, a person who is not clinically obese or even overweight according to the BMI may consider herself fat because she no longer fits into the clothes she used to wear, while someone who has been corpulent all her life may not consider herself 'fat', even if others do, because it is a state of embodiment to which she has become accustomed. Even in the clinical setting, fatness is dependent on the context. Someone with a BMI of 35 (and thus categorized as 'obese') who enters a general practitioner's surgery would very probably be advised to lose weight, whereas an individual who has gone from a BMI of 65 ('extremely obese') to 35 due to gastric band surgery is considered by his surgeon to be no longer in need of intervention. Not only does such an individual consider himself much slimmer, his surgeon, who is accustomed to seeing and treating very obese patients, also considers him 'normal' or simply 'overweight, like a lot of people' and therefore acceptably rather than 'dangerously' fat (Throsby 2012: 6). Some critics claim, indeed, that all individuals have internalized 'fat-phobic self-hatred' to the extent that even thin people are not entirely satisfied with their body size, or feel the continual need to discipline their bodies in order to remain thin, and that most people 'feel fat' at some times in their lives (Mitchell 2005; Burgard *et al.* 2009: 337; Wann 2009).

Challenging 'obesity'

Critical scholarship and fat activism have been further influenced by political movements centred on identity politics and the challenging of medical dominance. One influential trend has been the growing scepticism more generally among members of the public about medicine and their willingness, at least among the more highly educated and members of the middle class, to challenge medical authority. The internet has played an important role here in providing alternative sources of medical information about health conditions, allowing people with similar conditions to join support groups and share information and experiences and providing an outlet for activists to critique medical knowledge and call for political action.

So too, the second-wave feminist movement, in its challenging of dominant discourses concerning women's bodies and its political activism, has been an extremely influential precursor to fat activism and critical scholarship. Indeed, the vast majority of fat activists are women who identify as feminists. Feminist scholars have been influential contributors to social analyses of the body, particularly in relation to concepts of femininity. In the 1980s and 1990s feminist writers produced books and articles about the social and cultural dimensions of eating disorders such as anorexia nervosa, bulimia nervosa and binge eating in relation to concepts of the ideal female body as thin. Since the turn of the century this focus has turned the production of critiques of the ways in which ideas about women's embodiment intersect with cultural concepts concerning fatness. Interestingly, both topics concern body size, ideals of feminine embodiment and the discipline of the body in relation to eating and exercise habits.

The gay or queer movement has also influenced fat activism and scholarly writings about fatness. Close parallels may be drawn in particular between fat studies/critical weight studies research and the sociocultural scholarship around HIV/AIDS. When HIV/AIDS emerged as a new medical condition in the early 1980s, because it was first manifested in gay men and linked to male-to-male sexual practices a framework of moralistic judgements grew around it, giving it meaning in both medical and lay understandings. To identify and critique these meanings and to make sense of the sociocultural dimensions of HIV/AIDS, a substantial body of research and writing by scholars working within the social sciences and humanities developed. Political activism was also an important part of critical scholarship on HIV/AIDS. Like fat activists, gay activists sought to challenge stigmatizing and moralistic discourses about the condition. In many ways, therefore, scholarship and cultural activism around HIV/AIDS, in concert with feminist scholarship and activism, have provided important antecedents upon which fat scholarship and activism has drawn.

A further social movement and area of academic inquiry that has many similarities with fat studies and critical weight studies is that of critical disability studies. The 'social model' of disability sees disability as a social construction. Proponents of this approach contend that people with certain limited body capacities or impairments that differ from the norm find themselves stigmatized and socially excluded, represented as inferior or lacking. Those who advocate the social model challenge this 'individual deficit' concept of disability and point to the limitations of the physical spaces, funding and support services offered to people with disabilities. They assert that it is society's inability to accommodate people who differ physically or intellectually from the norm which is the source of their 'disability'. Disability activists have therefore agitated for better services and support for people with disabilities, while the academic field of critical disability studies has examined the social and cultural dimensions of disability. As I will discuss in greater detail later in this book, some writers on fat embodiment have contended that fatness should be viewed as a disability, and employed some of the theoretical arguments from critical disability studies to make this claim.

Chapter outline

In Chapter 2 I provide an overview of various ways of 'thinking about fat', including the anti-obesity perspective, the critical biomedical perspective, the libertarian perspective, ethical approaches, critical weight studies/fat studies and fat activism. The significant theorists who have been employed in socio-cultural analyses of fat will be introduced, thus providing the theoretical background for the discussions in the remainder of the book. Chapter 3 addresses the regulation of bodies in the context of obesity discourse. The discussion draws particularly upon the Foucauldian concepts of governmentality, biopower and biopolitics to explain how medical and public health discourses contribute to a view of the body as requiring discipline, monitoring and surveillance to identify and prevent obesity. Chapter 4 looks at the moral meanings underpinning contemporary notions of fatness as well as the ways in which the fat body is considered grotesque and transgressive and may provoke deep and intense feelings of disgust. I argue in this chapter that the fat body challenges hegemonic notions of embodied containment and control and thus is threatening to the social order. In Chapter 5 I examine the embodied experience of fatness: how it feels to be and feel fat. The discussion draws on empirical data from studies interviewing fat people as well as fat scholars' own writings on the experience of fatness and material from weight-loss blogs. Chapter 6 examines the fat activist movement and its accompanying politics and discourses surrounding the fat body. This chapter also reviews debates in the feminist literature concerning size acceptance politics. The book finishes with some brief concluding comments concerning whether it may be contended that the power of obesity discourse has begun to dissipate, the nature and source of resistance to this discourse and a review of the overarching themes underpinning the discussions throughout the book.

2

THINKING ABOUT FAT

A review of different perspectives

There are various perspectives circulating about fat bodies in the expert, popular and academic literature. The most well known, the 'anti-obesity' perspective, argues that fatness is a significant health and social problem which must urgently be treated and prevented. Yet a number of other perspectives have emerged which challenge this view for various reasons. After a brief review of the anti-obesity position, the remainder of the chapter addresses these different critical stances on fat, including discussion of the critical biomedical, libertarian, ethical, critical weight studies/fat studies and fat activism perspectives.

The anti-obesity perspective

Those researching and writing within the anti-obesity perspective – mainly including academics, policy makers, politicians and practitioners from within medicine, nutrition and public health areas such as epidemiology and health promotion, but also some

researchers in the social sciences – tend to take an unpro-
blematized approach to fat. For them, fatness – or what they
prefer to term 'overweight' or 'obesity', or sometimes 'excess
body weight' – is a major health risk for those who are designated as being overweight or obese, associated with such significant health problems as cardiovascular heart disease, diabetes
and early death. This perspective contends that the numbers of
people who are overweight and obese are rapidly increasing to
an unprecedented level in many countries, both western and
developing. Hence the common use of the term 'obesity
epidemic' in this literature, or even the neologism 'globesity', to
denote the spread of the epidemic around the world.

Anti-obesity writers and practitioners assert that something
must be done urgently about the increasing prevalence of
obesity, because of the health risks they have identified as
associated with this body type. They call for people who are
overweight or obese to lose weight so as to avoid becoming ill
by engaging in preventive strategies such as taking more exercise
and reducing food consumption. As the foreword to a recent
British government report entitled *Healthy Lives, Healthy People:
A Call to Action on Obesity in England* put it:

> Overweight and obesity are a direct consequence of eating
> and drinking more calories and using up too few. We need
> to be honest with ourselves and recognize that we need to
> make some changes to control our weight. Increasing
> physical activity is important but, for most of us who are
> overweight and obese, eating and drinking less is key to
> weight loss.
>
> *(Department of Health 2011: 3)*

The anti-obesity discourse is very familiar because of the high
level of attention it has received in popular forums such as the
news media, television documentaries and reality series, books,
magazines and websites directed at health and weight issues and

advertising for weight-loss products, as well as in statements from governmental officials and in health promotion campaigns. The 'obesity epidemic' has been publicized untiringly in news media reports in countries such as the United States, the United Kingdom and Australia since the late 1990s, when the scientific reports about obesity began to become more urgent and insistent about the threat posed by obesity to the public's health and the health system. The news media responded to these reports by publishing related accounts in increasing numbers. Numerous news stories made reference to the 'obesity epidemic', the 'obesity crisis' and the 'war on obesity', echoing the phraseology of medical and public health experts and policy makers. They were thus central in conveying the meanings of catastrophe and threat concerning the risks of obesity to their audiences (Lupton 2004; Gard and Wright 2005; Boero 2007; Saguy and Almeling 2008; Holland *et al.* 2011).

Researchers within the anti-obesity perspective have conducted studies seeking to identify the 'risk factors' for obesity, the physiological processes by which obesity occurs, the genetic causes of obesity, medical, behavioural and dietary solutions and the statistical relationship between body weight and various diseases and conditions such as elevated blood pressure, type II diabetes and cardiovascular disease as well as early mortality. Public health researchers have directed their attention at identifying 'at risk' groups, producing statistical 'maps' of geographical areas or tables of social groups to determine which have larger numbers of people who are overweight or obese. Social scientists have sought to identify the social underpinnings leading to behaviours believed to cause fatness, such as eating the wrong foods or lack of exercise, or the social groups most 'at risk' and the reasons why they may be more susceptible to overweight and obesity as well as locate the geographical areas in which 'high-risk' groups live.

As a result of such research and subsequent claims about the prevalence, causes and effects of obesity, many high-powered and well-funded organizations have been established in various countries as well as internationally, including the International Association for the Study of Obesity and the International Obesity Task Force. A plethora of health education campaigns have been funded in many countries to educate populations about the risks of obesity and encourage those deemed to be at risk to lose weight, including the 'Let's Move' campaign in the United States, the British 'Change4Life' campaign and the 'Measure Up?' and 'Swap It, Don't Stop It' campaigns in Australia.

Much of the anti-obesity discourse directs responsibility for weight control at the individual. Nevertheless, there is also a perspective within anti-obesity arguments that takes a more social structuralist approach to obesity by identifying some socioeconomic reasons for the increase in overweight and obesity rates. Some anti-obesity experts refer to an 'obesogenic environment', or an environment in which obesity is facilitated: for example, by the sheer abundance of cheap, poor-quality and high kilojoule foods, proliferation of fast food outlets and advertising for such food, the entry of women into the workforce, resulting in fewer healthy home-cooked meals, the greater propensity of children and young people to engage in sedentary pursuits such as television watching and computer games and the increasing physical immobility of people due to contemporary working and transport conditions. These structural factors identified as contributing to obesity are very difficult to challenge or change as they form part of a complex network of agribusiness, the processing, marketing and distribution of food as well as major social changes relating to working and everyday life. Nonetheless, various consumer lobby groups and policy makers have subsequently called for the government to develop greater restrictions on the activities of 'Big Food', such as junk-food advertising controls, provide more cycle paths and parks for people to exercise in, change the food offered to children in school canteens and so on.

The concern about the rapid spread of obesity around the world, including in developing countries, also reflects anxieties about globalization, the decline of traditional habits and modernization. Discourses on globesity argue that traditional eating habits have been corrupted by modernization and globalization, leading to wealth among the few and poverty among the many. The 'traditional culture' in these representations is positioned as that of the 'noble savage', healthy in its state of nature, which is now being contaminated by 'civilization' (Gilman 2010). In non-western countries, discourses on obesity often tend to position 'the west' broadly, or more specifically the United States, as contaminating traditional ethnic cultures and spreading fatness. In China, for example, obesity is seen to be the result of the 'westernization' of Chinese society, including the importation of unhealthy western foods replacing what was seen to be the traditional 'healthy' Chinese diet. Discourses on obesity in China thus bespeak concerns about the rapid changes in Chinese society, leading to the degeneration of traditional morals and mores in response to the invasion from the west of lifestyle habits (Gilman 2010).

Critical perspectives

There are a range of perspectives which have sought to challenge the anti-obesity approach, with varying theoretical and political standpoints.

The critical biomedical perspective

Directly challenging this dominant discourse on its own grounds – that is, asserting counter-claims drawn from analysing the medico-scientific and epidemiological literature – are those commentators I have grouped together under the rubric of the 'critical biomedical perspective'. They include writers from a number of disciplines, especially the social sciences, but few from within medicine and public health themselves.

Prominent writers from the critical biomedical camp include the Americans Glen Gaesser, an exercise physiologist who wrote *Big Fat Lies: The Truth About Your Weight and Your Health* (2002), Paul Campos, a legal academic and author of *The Obesity Myth: Why America's Obsession with Weight is Hazardous to Your Health* (2004) and J. Eric Oliver, a political scientist who penned *Fat Politics: The Real Story Behind America's Obesity Epidemic* (2006). Although these three writers chose to direct their books largely at a popular audience, their contentions have also been published in respected medical and scientific publications such as *New Scientist* and the *International Journal of Epidemiology* and as chapters in academic books (see, for example, Campos *et al.* 2006; Campos 2011). These authors seek to demonstrate that the anti-obesity position depends on the poor interpretation of data or over-generalization, and use evidence from alternative scientific sources to argue that their own scientific claims are more 'accurate' or 'true' than are those of the anti-obesity group. They contend that the findings of anti-obesity research are 'pseudofindings promulgated as fact' and 'based on very shaky evidence', as Oliver (2006: x) puts it.

The following is a summary of the main arguments put forward by writers in the critical biomedical perspective:

- It is not the case that there are far greater numbers of fat people now compared to several decades ago. While there has been a modest increase in average weight, this does not represent an 'epidemic of obesity'.
- Life expectancy in western countries has risen, not fallen, despite alleged growing rates of obesity and the supposed life-threatening health conditions caused by obesity.
- There is no statistical evidence that being fat necessarily equates to a greater risk of ill health or disease. Statistics show that only those people at the extreme end of the weight spectrum (the 'morbidly obese' in medical terminology)

demonstrate negative health effects from their weight. The data show that higher body weight may even be protective of health in older people.

- The epidemiological literature has been unable to demonstrate that significant weight loss improves fat people's health status. Indeed continual attempts by fat people to lose weight can actually be negative to their health status if it involves extreme diets, being caught in a cycle of losing and gaining weight or poor dietary habits.
- Fatness is often a symptom rather than the cause of ill health and disease.
- Cardiovascular fitness and regular physical activity are more important for good health than body weight.

Given these criticisms of anti-obesity discourse, writers within the critical biomedical perspective call for public health focus to be on a 'healthy lifestyle' involving regular exercise and a nutritious diet, rather than on weight loss itself. They are equally as passionate in propounding their theories about health and physical fitness as are anti-obesity researchers and policy advocates about weight loss. Such writers still, therefore, operate within the biomedical paradigm, but prefer one set of scientific findings over others (Gard and Wright 2005).

Several of these writers do, however, go on to identify what they see as the political dimensions of the obesity epidemic discourse. They contend that many of the researchers from the anti-obesity perspective make their allegedly unsubstantiated claims because they are being funded by pharmaceutical and other companies producing weight-loss products, their assertions allow them to win substantial research grants or because they are members of policy agencies which can then can claim higher budgets to deal with the 'obesity crisis'. According to Oliver (2006: 6), for example, 'The very same people who have proclaimed that obesity is a major health problem also stand the most to gain from it being classified as a disease'.

Campos (2004: xvii) is even more extreme in his assertions, contending that some researchers and policy advocates espousing 'obesity propaganda' are making their claims based on pecuniary interests, and that they are deliberately misleading the public to achieve these interests. He further asserts that these experts are engaged in deliberate discrimination and 'bigotry' to render fat people 'social pariahs'. As this suggests, the terminology used by many of these critics is sometimes as extreme and generalizing as those offered by the anti-obesity proponents.

There are also a small number of iconoclastic nutritionists writing in the sceptical academic literature who have challenged the science of obesity. These critics have called for other nutrition researchers and dieticians to relinquish their intense focus on losing weight by dieting. They call instead for an approach that recognizes that health may be achieved across a diverse range of body sizes. Like the critics referred to above, these radical nutritionists focus on physical fitness and healthy eating as the main components of good health rather than body weight per se (Aphramor 2005; Aphramor and Gringas 2008, 2011).

It is not the intention of this book to evaluate the claims and counter-claims of the anti-obesity versus the sceptical position, as this has been achieved effectively and in detail elsewhere (see the writers referred to above as well as Gard and Wright 2005; Gard 2011). Rather, my aim is to highlight that legitimate challenges to the dominant paradigm of obesity science exist and that these need to be considered as part of understanding the cultural response to fatness in contemporary western societies. It is interesting to note that despite the accumulating body of literature produced by the dissenting views of the critical biomedical perspective, for the most part their arguments have yet to be fully acknowledged or debated by the anti-obesity camp or in the mass media. These influential sources of authority continue for the large part to assert the views of the anti-obesity perspective as unchallenged.

Libertarian sceptics

The writers referred to above tend to present a liberal political view by critiquing the vested interests of the weight-loss industry, for example, in promoting the anti-obesity argument. Ironically, therefore, their assertions have been taken up by conservative organizations and right-wing groups such as the US Center for Consumer Freedom, a coalition of restaurants, food companies and consumers who have united to fight against notions that people should cut down their eating in the interests of their health because they see their profits threatened. Such groups argue against government intervention into eating habits and food advertising, advocating, instead, personal responsibility, autonomy and consumer choice over regulation (Halse 2009; Herrick 2009). These organizations and individuals, therefore, comprise another sceptical group, one emerging from the commercial perspective which is reluctant to relinquish customers for their products. The industry sceptics often conveniently fail to position themselves as industry lobbyists with their own commercial interests to defend (Gard 2011).

Sceptics from industry are joined by libertarian political advocates, often writing from within right-wing or free-market think tanks in the United States and the United Kingdom, who disdain what they see as the 'nanny state' attempting to impose its views upon its citizens. Some writers in this camp, such as those contributing to the book *Diet Nation: Exposing the Obesity Crusade* (Basham *et al.* 2006), even go so far as to represent anti-obesity advocates as 'socialists' working against the appropriate forces of capitalism (Gard 2010). For this latter group, attempts by the state to persuade citizens to lose weight via health promotion campaigns or interventions in doctors' surgeries or to legislate to lessen the effects of the 'obesogenic' environment, by controlling the sale of certain food products in schools, for example, are viewed as restrictive of individuals' freedom and autonomy. Although they may adopt the assertions of the critical biomedical sceptics to use as support for their contentions, they are not directly involved in challenging the science of obesity (Gard 2010).

Ethical challenges

Quite apart from the debate concerning the validity of obesity science, some medical and public health ethicists have raised the question of the ethics of anti-obesity campaigns and programmes. They assert that the intense focus on people's body weight contravenes human rights: in particular, the right to dignity which is breached by health promotion campaigns or advertising for exercise services or weight-control products directed at stigmatizing or making fun of fat people. They point out that fat people are also commonly subjected to discrimination and ill treatment based on their appearance, attacks on their privacy and reputation and coercion in the interests of losing weight (see also Chapter 5), all of which contravene human rights protocols.

Writers critical of the ethical issues around weight control claim that the obligation of medicine and public health to preserve dignity, privacy and treat everyone equally, and to 'do no harm', is regularly undermined by the ways in which fat people are treated and portrayed. They question to what extent unwanted paternalistic intervention into the lives of fat people, their positioning as responsible for their body weight and attempts to persuade them to change their habits in the interests of losing weight are justified, particularly if these interventions result in continual cycles of dieting and weight regain and feelings of guilt and shame in fat people (Holm 2007; Puhl and Heuer 2010; O'Hara and Gregg 2012).

Critical weight studies/fat studies

As I observed in the previous chapter, the emergence of the 'obesity epidemic' has resulted in a response from scholars and researchers in the humanities and social sciences that has produced many interesting analyses of the social, historical, cultural and political dimensions of fat embodiment and obesity discourse. Several of these writers position themselves in 'critical weight' or 'critical obesity studies', while others prefer the term 'fat studies', and still others, although sharing similar concerns and foci, may not label themselves as belonging to either.

Several social scientists have engaged in detailed critiques of the medical and public health research and policy documents about obesity. Like the writers within the critical biomedical perspective, they have called attention to the use of alarmist rhetoric in this literature which blows statistics out of proportion, the frequent generalizing of one set of data from a specific social group or country to another, the dubious assumptions that are made in the reports, the transformation of complex data into overly simplified and therefore misleading 'facts' and the transforming of speculative idea into scientific fact. However these social scientists tend not to claim that medical and public health researchers and health professionals are corrupt or self-serving, deliberately seeking to put forward false statistics to mislead the general public for their own interests, as do many of the writers directing their critique towards a more general readership (as well as some fat activist writers). Rather, they seek to identify the scientific uncertainties, complexities and contradictions in this literature, adopting a sociological approach by attempting to identify the underlying assumptions which shape obesity researchers' conclusions about their work (Gard and Wright 2005; Gard 2009, 2010, 2011; Monaghan 2005a; Jutel 2006; see also further discussion of this position in Chapter 3).

Researchers across the social sciences and humanities, including sociology, critical social psychology, anthropology, critical geography, philosophy and literary studies and the interdisciplinary fields of gender studies, cultural studies, media studies and queer studies, have developed a valuable literature elucidating the cultural meanings of fat embodiment. They have investigated the lived experience of being fat, predominantly using the technique of indepth interviews or focus groups. They have also engaged in textual analyses, using such texts as policy documents, health promotion materials, television programmes, exercise videos, literature, theatre, magazine and newspaper articles and film to identify the ways in which fat embodiment is portrayed and the dominant meanings conveyed to audiences of such texts. Some have engaged in detailed critiques of obesity science, as noted above. Many have adopted a poststructuralist perspective to identify the political dimensions and power relations inherent in the ways fat people are treated in contemporary western societies.

Michel Foucault's writings on the body, the medical clinic and the medical gaze, biopower and biopolitics in contemporary neoliberal societies have been particularly influential in the scholarship on fat in the humanities and social sciences (Foucault 1973, 1988, 1991). The terms 'biopower' and 'biopolitics' refer to how power relations are produced and reproduced in the context of human bodies. From this perspective, medical and public health researchers and practitioners play an important role in the defining, regulation and surveilling of bodies, pronouncing on what should be considered 'normal' and what should be considered liable to expert intervention. Foucault's analysis of the medical gaze as it constitutes and disciplines patients' bodies is related in the critical literature to the ways in which medical discourses prescribe the 'proper' weight and size of bodies and define certain bodies – including fat bodies – as pathological and others as normal.

Foucault's writings on governmentality and neoliberalism have been taken up by writers in critical weight studies/fat studies who have examined the discourses and practices of public health as it constructs and then addresses the 'problem of obesity' in populations. The techniques of governmentality are associated with normalization, or the establishment of disciplines, knowledges and technologies that serve to proffer advice on how individuals should conduct themselves and deport their bodies. Foucault's concept of 'the practices of the self' has also been adopted to explore the ways in which health-related imperatives are part of the construction of the entrepreneurial subject that is privileged in neoliberal societies. Practices of the self include the ways in which individuals act on their bodies and selves to achieve happiness, fulfilment and self-actualization. Governmentality incorporates both these practices of the self and the more apparent forms of external government, such as health promotional directives, that are carried out by state agencies or other institutions for strategic ends. These directives are internalized by individuals and then practised (or resisted) as part of their efforts to achieve the ideal of being a 'good', 'productive' and 'healthy' citizen.

The work of the sociologist Erving Goffman (1963) has also been employed by some scholars to understand the stigmatizing dimensions of fat embodiment. Goffman wrote about how the reaction of other people 'spoils' an individual's identity if those reactions are negative, demonstrating severe disapproval or repugnance. These reactions, resulting in social stigma, may be incited by what is perceived to be difference from the norm or a form of physical deformity. Social stigma resulting in a 'spoilt identity' creates a division between Self and Other, and has repercussions for the stigmatized individual in his or her dealings in social life such as exclusion, marginalization, ostracism, social discrimination and less access to privileged occupations, housing, educational opportunities and so on. Social stigma may thus cause both emotional distress and socioeconomic disadvantage. The relevance of this work on social stigma is clear in the ways in which fat people are subjected to abuse, humiliation and shaming practices and are portrayed in both medical and popular forums as sick, irresponsible, ignorant and abnormal.

The French philosopher Marcel Merleau-Ponty's work on embodied being is relevant to understanding the ways in which fat people experience living their bodies. Merleau-Ponty (1962, 1968) emphasizes how subjectivity (concepts of selfhood) is always inevitably experienced via embodiment. Despite the dominant belief in western thought that the mind and body are separate from each other, Merleau-Ponty argues that we can never completely escape our fleshly selves. Our 'being-in-the-world', or our lived experience, is always embodied and always in interaction with others' bodies. Thus, the ways in which others interact with us, touch us, view us, are essential parts of our 'being-in-the-world'. In the context of fat embodiment, this approach to the body and the self recognizes that they are not fixed or essential, but rather are in a state of flux, depending upon the other people with whom people are interacting. Scholars within cultural studies and sociology have adopted this perspective to examine the lived experiences of being fat.

Deleuze and Guattari (1985, 1988), also French philosophers, add the important context of space as part of their theorizing of the body. They have developed the concept of the 'assemblage' to articulate the ways in which bodies interact with other bodies but also with discourses, practices, material objects, non-human living organisms and space and place. The concept therefore goes beyond a preoccupation with language which is often a feature of poststructuralist theorizing and research to emphasizing the role played by material objects in shaping selves and bodies. Deleuze and Guattari also use the concept of 'territories', which describes features of space and place and the interactions of humans and non-humans that take place within, through and between them. Here again, the fluidity and dynamic nature of embodiment as it is conceptualized and experienced is emphasized. Critical geographers, in particular, have adopted these concepts of assemblages and territories to explore the spatial dimensions of fat embodiment, but they have also begun to be adopted in sociological research on weight control, particularly in relation to children and young people.

Feminist philosophers have also proved extremely influential in fat scholarship, particularly given the dominance of feminist writers on the body in general. The work of Elizabeth Grosz (1994, 1995), for example, is frequently used by feminist scholars to explicate the underlying meanings of female embodiment, including fat female bodies. So too, Julia Kristeva's (1982) work on abjection and Margit Shildrick's (1997) writings on 'leaky bodies' have direct implications for theorizing fat embodiment. All three point to the symbolic cultural meanings given to female embodiment which emphasize the fluidities of the female body, its lack of containment and its tendency to leak, both metaphorically and literally. They identify the ways in which the fat female body (and, by implication, the feminized male fat body) are positioned as symbolically Other to the Self. They argue that the leakiness and permeability of female embodiment, both literal and figurative, challenge the dominant western ideals of containment and control of the body/self. As such, women's bodies are culturally represented and viewed as inferior, lacking and constantly in danger of invoking disgust. They are Other to the ideal of the tight, contained and controlled body of the middle-class white man.

Queer theory, itself heavily influenced by feminist theory, has also been taken up by some scholars in critical weight studies/fat studies analyses. This approach has been particularly influential in literary studies, cultural studies and fat activist writings on fat identity and embodiment. Queer theory originated from scholars wanting to critically address the cultural construction of sexual identity, gender and sexual desire, with a particular interest in gay, lesbian, bisexual and transgender identities and how these are marginalized in mainstream society (see, for example, Butler 1990; Sedgwick 1990). 'Queer' is now often defined more expansively as referring to all individuals or social groups who challenge normativity. In such analyses, to 'queer' a topic such as fat embodiment is to challenge dominant, taken-for-granted meanings around that topic and identify the power relations inherent within and perpetuated by these meanings, particularly those which seek to categorize some groups as 'normal' and others as 'deviant'. Queer theory attempts to both identify and deconstruct these meanings, to make them visible rather than latent, and to subvert them by challenging or resisting them. Queer theory also sees identities as unstable and dynamic rather than fixed. Queer theorists argue that such identities as gender, sexual identity and fatness are performative and fluid rather than an essentialist part of subjectivity, and thus are open to change and contestation.

Fat activism

Not all of those scholars in critical weight studies/fat studies would necessarily define themselves as activists. Rather, they may well position themselves as critics or researchers who are dispassionately analysing the sociocultural meanings of fatness. Fat activism, in contrast, is explicitly and passionately political, directed at social justice and the ending of discrimination against fat people. Fat activists use a variety of terms – fat pride, fat acceptance, size acceptance – to convey their dominant aim: to challenge and reframe the prevailing negative meanings around the fat body, so as to render fat bodies visible, powerful, healthy and positive. 'We smash stereotypes. We explode the ideas that fat women are victims or that girls have to be skinny in order to get a boyfriend or that fat chicks gotta wear muumuus. We are happy and fat – most of the time' (Mitchell 2005: 217).

The emotional dimensions of fat embodiment are stated more loudly, clearly and often very eloquently in the writings of those who identify themselves as fat activists than in other critical literature: in particular the humiliation, frustration and anger they feel at being marginalized and positioned as pathological, lazy and lacking self-discipline, as well as a certain ambivalence about fat embodiment in some cases. Many writers from this perspective highlight what they see as the broader political and economic aspects of the current focus on controlling people's body weight, claiming, like several of the sceptics referred to above, that the government, the medical profession, the pharmaceutical industry, advertising companies and the weight-loss industry exaggerate the ill-effects of fatness to make money or pursue personal ambitions. They argue that it is not fatness itself that causes ill health, but rather the negative social attitudes and portrayals of fat people that lead to their marginalization, shaming and the kinds of discrimination which mean that they are more likely to be socially and economically disadvantaged.

There are resonances in fat activism with the contentions of activists in the feminist, black, gay and lesbian and disability rights movements, in which the marginalization of and discrimination against women, black people, gays and lesbians and people with disabilities, based on their physical characteristics and the negative cultural associations of these characteristics, have been identified and trenchantly challenged. These movements, based as they are on identity politics, require the identification of their members with the stigmatization and discrimination they seek to uncover and redress. They draw upon the long-harboured resentment, anger and frustration of members of their movements to inspire the action required to instigate social change.

Fat activists are overwhelmingly women who adopt a feminist perspective on fat embodiment and who themselves identify as fat. Some of these individuals have written popular books and blogs about fat discrimination and fat politics, and many such activists are involved in support groups and events which attempt to highlight discrimination issues, agitate for legislation against discrimination of fat people and present positive representations of fat bodies, mostly in relation to female fat embodiment. Some of these accounts are atheoretical and do not engage with the academic literature on fat embodiment. However many fat activists also employ the perspectives and theories offered by the social sciences and humanities and several are themselves academics, seeking to disseminate their critiques to a scholarly rather than a popular audience (for example, Solovay and Rothblum 2009; Cooper 1997, 2009, 2010; Murray 2005, 2008, 2009a, 2009b).

3

GOVERNING FAT BODIES

Fat bodies have become the target of a vast network of surveillance, monitoring and regulating strategies and technologies emerging from state-sponsored authorities, medical expertise and commercial enterprises. This chapter looks at the ways in which fat bodies are governed via these strategies and technologies, including the assumptions, tacit knowledges and power relations which underpin them.

Medical power and the 'obesity epidemic'

Medicine and public health are intertwined authoritative institutions which have been immensely influential in the ways in which individuals understand, perceive and experience their bodies. Medical discourses and practices are directed at individual bodies in the context of the clinical setting, while public health takes up medical knowledge to focus on the health of population groups. Both institutions have been integral to the construction of the 'obesity epidemic' and in advising on how people should conduct their everyday lives in the quest to control their weight to 'normal' levels in the interests of their health. As this suggests, while medical and public health knowledges and practices are largely considered benevolent and free of ideology, they often have unintended consequences which reinforce underlying assumptions about fatness.

I would not argue, as some of the more controversial fat activists and obesity sceptics have done, that medical and public health experts are deliberately attempting to stigmatize fat people, engaging in 'fat genocide' by attempting to encourage fat people to lose weight, or that such experts bear a conscious hatred of fat people and are attempting to further their own careers at fat people's expense (although perhaps there may be a tiny minority for whom this is true). The operation of power in medicine and public health is far more subtle, diffuse and complex than that. The 'anti-obesity' position, and all its associated claims, research, commodities, practices, discourses and meanings, is a complex social movement comprised of many social actors, groups and organizations ranging across a range of sites, from the education system, the family, academia, government, mass media and commodity culture (Gard and Wright 2005; Gard 2011).

Medicine and public health are situated within a cultural context in which certain long-held beliefs and assumptions about certain kinds of bodies circulate. Like other powerful institutions, medicine and public health draw upon, reproduce and sometimes emphasize these beliefs and assumptions in ways of which the practitioners and researchers engaged in these institutions are often unaware (Lupton 1995, 2012; Petersen and Lupton 1996). Thus, in the case of fatness, medical practitioners and public health researchers and policy exponents have tended to unquestioningly take up various belief systems and discourses which give meaning to fat bodies, just as do the mass media, the education system and lay people, including many fat people themselves.

By virtue of their authority as the ultimate knowledge producers on matters to do with health and the body, bolstered by the credence given to apparently neutral free scientific research and statistics, however, the pronouncements of medicine and public health on fat bear more legitimacy than any other knowledge source. Despite experts' pronouncements of certainty many aspects of the causes and consequences of overweight and obesity are poorly understood by scientists and medical researchers (Gard and Wright 2005; Gard 2011). In making their claims, these experts are drawing on beliefs that are seen to be commonsense and self-evident, based on centuries of dominant understandings about how the body works and how health is maintained, as well as more recent anxieties about the dangers of technology, particularly in relation to children (Gard and Wright 2005; Monaghan 2005a; Jutel 2006, 2009).

The social construction of 'overweight' and 'obesity'

As I noted in Chapter 2, some critics have contended that the use of the medical term 'obesity' in itself serves to medicalize fat embodiment, bringing it into the sphere of medical treatment as problematic: as a disease or precursor to disease. Obesity is classified as a chronic disease by the World Health Organization. Thus if an individual is defined as obese according to the BMI, then he or she is viewed as being automatically ill, regardless of his or her actual state of health (Ross 2005: 95). Yet concepts of 'fat', 'overweight' or 'obesity' are all arbitrary social categories, defined in different ways in different historical, social and cultural settings. Indeed the category of 'overweight' is often conflated with 'obese' in expert and popular discourses.

Decisions about how much body fat is too much, and what kind of body fat is risky (located on the abdomen or other sites on the body, for example) are subject to a high degree of contention, dispute or uncertainty within the biomedical literature (Gard and Wright 2005; Ross 2005; Evans et al. 2008). As Ross (2005: 92) points out:

the problem with defining obesity is deciding what is excessive. How much adipose tissue do we need? How fat is obese? What are the advantages and disadvantages of being fat? And how fat do we have to be to be personally disadvantaged or a burden on society? Or how fat do we have to be to be classified as ill?

While in the past the medical literature often described fatness as pathological, it was not until the 2000s that overweight (as opposed to obesity) became a clinical entity in itself. Where once the term 'overweight' was used predominantly as an adjective to refer to a sign or a symptom, by the 2000s it appeared more frequently to describe a condition or disease in itself, with its own set of symptoms and treatment strategies and requirements for prevention. Like obesity, therefore, over-weight became medicalized as a medical condition. A number of factors came together to pathologize overweight: the assumption that the physical appearance of the body denotes the nature of the individual; the generalized ability to measure fatness using an 'objective' scientific instrument such as a set of scales or the BMI; the privileging of quantitative measurement and statistical analysis in biomedicine; and the value of medicine as a rhetorical strategy in promoting commodities directed at weight loss (Jutel 2006, 2009).

Defining obesity as a disease has resulted in a plethora of medical treatments to 'treat' this disease, including specialist doctors who focus on prescribing pharmaceutical solutions for weight loss or engage in weight-loss surgical techniques. Some critics have asserted that the pathologizing of fatness as 'over-weight' or 'obesity' renders those who have been classified as such vulnerable to the persuasions of commercial enterprises attempting to sell weight-reduction commodities, such as phar-maceuticals, and special dietary aids (Murray 2009a; Jutel 2009; Wann 2009). It is certainly the case that there is a massive weight-loss industry which is devoted to appealing to the vulnerabilities, anxieties and fears of people who have been medically classified as overweight or obese, or who have defined themselves as 'too fat'.

Various measurements and assessment technologies are employed by state and other organizations to scrutinize bodies and identify the 'normal' from the 'pathological' in relation to body weight. These technologies include scales, height charts, tape measurements, pedometers, workout machines, dietary guidelines, fitness videos, computer games such as Wii that incorporate health and fitness activities, diet pills and special dietary foods, medically prescribed weight-loss drugs, apps for smartphones and tablet computers and at the most extreme and highly technological, weight-loss surgery. They configure a certain type of bodily assemblage which is constituted around the imperatives of anti-obesity discourse as well as the inducements of commodity culture concerning the attractiveness of the slim body.

The concept of assemblages as it is used in relation to health education in populations brings together the Foucauldian concept of the government of the body with that of the Deleuze and Guattarian assemblages: 'governmental assemblages' as Leahy (2009: 173) puts it. This continual and interactive process of constructing such an assemblage produces categories of bodies – the fat body, the normal body – which are then treated in different ways depending on how they are categorized. In their digitalized formats, in which various forms of data are collated to produce categories, bodily measurements are abstracted from the socioeconomic context in which these bodies live by reducing the complexities of this context to easily measurable and readily collated statistics (Rich et al. 2011).

The BMI and defining 'obesity'

The BMI used by orthodox medicine to measure, standardize and categorize body weight, including defining overweight and obesity versus 'normality', has been the subject of trenchant critique from various brands of obesity sceptic. The BMI is used as a measurement across a wide range of contexts: in the doctor's surgery, in public health surveillance attempts to measure levels of overweight and obesity across a population, in health promotion campaigns, in schools, by insurance companies, weight-loss companies, gyms, in popular media accounts of body weight, as a criterion for entry into the armed forces and so on. It uses an individual's weight and height to calculate a figure which supposedly indicates how fat that person is. The argument for this measure is that body weight alone does not provide an indication of whether an individual is 'normal' or 'underweight' or 'overweight', as there are large variations of height across a population. One would reasonably assume that a very tall person, for example, would weigh more than a very short person. The BMI, therefore, measures body mass using both weight and height. A person's weight is divided by that individual's height squared to calculate the BMI. The resultant BMI is then compared against a chart which gives guidelines for underweight, normal weight, overweight and obesity. If an individual's BMI falls within the 'overweight' or 'obese' categories, she or he is then defined as 'at-risk' from the diseases associated with excess body weight and as having a defined medical condition which requires medical intervention or lifestyle change.

The influence and extent of use of the BMI is such that it has been contended that it was a major factor in making the 'obesity epidemic' possible, because it provided the opportunity to classify individuals and to statistically measure body mass across population groups, allowing for comparisons between different groups based on physical location, gender, age, social class, ethnicity and so on (Halse 2009). Yet what is often ignored or glossed over in expert and popular representations and uses of the BMI is the fact that it is an arbitrary figure. The cut-off point for overweight on the BMI scale was lowered by the

National Institutes of Health in the United States in 1998, resulting in many more individuals being designated as overweight even though their body weight had not actually changed (Halse 2009; Wann 2009). The 'obesity epidemic' rests on these changing figures, which inflated the numbers of individuals being designated as overweight.

Critics also point out that the BMI is an inaccurate means of measuring body weight in relation to height, as it does not allow for variation between people based on their body frame or relative muscularity, nor for age and gender. It measures body mass, not body fat. On its own, it is no indication of whether an individual is in good health or not or at risk from ill health. It is not a useful measure for children and does not make allowances for differences between ethnic groups (Gard and Wright 2005; Evans and Colls 2009). The scientific aura surrounding the BMI, its constant use as a measure of relative body weight across medicine and public health authorities and its mathematical formula all give the BMI apparent validity and trustworthiness as an objective fact that is devoid of subjective value, and which is therefore difficult to dispute. Yet the BMI is far from value-free in its meaning and use. Once individuals are deemed to be 'overweight' or 'obese' by the BMI, they then become the subject of efforts to persuade them to change their lives in order to lose weight and become 'normal'. The BMI thus acts as a regulating, disciplining and normalizing body metric, making distinctions between 'the normal' and 'the pathological' which bear with them moral meanings and judgements (Gard and Wright 2005; Evans *et al.* 2008; Evans and Colls 2009; Halse 2009).

Biopolitics and personal responsibility for body weight

For those writing about the government of the body, the concepts of biopolitics, biopower and the bio-citizen are all central.

Each one of these concepts emerges from Foucault's writings on the state's relationship to citizens in the context of neoliberal politics. As Foucault (1991) argued, neoliberal governments depend upon their citizens adopting their injunctions voluntarily, rather than relying on coercive or punitive approaches to maintaining social order and facilitating prosperity. His writings on the care of the self (Foucault 1988) also emphasize the importance of individual bodily management as part of conforming to the notion of the well-regulated citizen who takes responsibility for her or his health and wellbeing. Such citizens are essential to the modern neoliberal state because they are productive and entrepreneurial. Their continued good health is required both because they contribute to the workings of the state as productive citizens and because they do not place an economic burden on the resources of the state by becoming ill and requiring health care. Hence the state's interest in monitoring and surveilling the health of its citizens at a population level, identifying 'at risk' subgroups for special attention, to ensure that citizens are doing the best they can to regulate their own bodies in the interests of maintaining good health (Lupton 1995, 1999; Petersen and Lupton 1996).

In the context of weight control, Foucauldian theoretical perspectives on the relationship between the state and the body/self can easily be adopted. Thus it may be argued that the imperatives on managing and reducing body weight that are articulated in government policy documents and state-sponsored health promotional materials are part of the apparatus of neoliberal state power that seeks to regulate, normalize and discipline its citizens to render them more productive. In doing so, neoliberal governments have mobilized resources from a plethora of medical, public health and social science experts, as well as drawing upon advertising and social marketing techniques in the attempt to publicize the risks associated with fatness.

It is clear that many influential forums, including medical and public health journals, policy documents, government-sponsored health promotion campaigns, news media reports and advertising for weight-loss products, portray body weight as an individual responsibility. It is asserted in these texts that it is up to individuals to recognize whether they are too fat and do something about it if they are. The British 'Change4Life' campaign, for example, had the explicit approach of positioning everyone as 'at risk' from obesity, calling for the whole population to examine their behaviour as part of recognizing that they may be already obese or engaging in lifestyle behaviours that would eventually lead to obesity (Evans *et al.* 2011).

In neoliberal societies the concept of 'free choice' is dominant. This concept presumes that consumer/citizens use their own assessment of risks and benefits when making choices about lifestyle commodities and behaviours. The government both supports free market enterprise and seeks to 'inform' citizens about the risks that may be associated with certain commodities. Thus there are highly established and profitable markets seeking to sell consumers products, such as fast foods and soft drinks, that are linked to overweight, as well as products directed at losing weight. In neoliberal societies, both are encouraged: it is considered up to consumer/citizens to make wise choices about which products they should buy and use as part of the project of self-actualization and fulfilment (Guthman and DuPuis 2006; Guthman 2009a). Ideal consumer/citizens, therefore, are able to continue to consume in a context of an abundance of tempting food but also to limit their consumption enough to demonstrate their capacity for self-discipline.

Because of this emphasis on personal responsibility for body weight and health status, people who have been given the label 'obese' are blamed for any illnesses they might develop, for it is regarded as a condition that is caused by lack of self-control and self-discipline. Some medical texts on obesity are overtly moralistic in their contentions that weight control is a matter of self-control and personal responsibility. They thus imply that fat people lack the necessary self-control and discipline to conform to standards of 'normal' weight. Murray (2009a: 81), for example, quotes an article published in the prestigious *Medical Journal of Australia* which proposes that a certain narrow BMI range should be nominated as a 'virtuous mean' to which individuals should aspire, and that staying within this range should be an ethical obligation of citizens.

Despite the emphasis in some policy and biomedical and public health documents on the social structural aspects of the environment in which people live which make it difficult to control body weight (the 'obesogenic environment'), the emphasis is still overwhelmingly on the individual's responsibility. The obesogenic perspective makes the simplistic assertion that because food is more readily available in contemporary societies people therefore consume more of it, and become fat. It assumes that the 'natural' state of the human body is to be thin (given the right environmental conditions) and that in this context of ready supply of poor quality food that all individuals may potentially become obese as they will be unable to resist the temptations or persuasions of over-eating or lack of exercise (Gard and Wright 2005; Colls and Evans 2009; Guthman 2009a; Rich and Evans 2009).

Governing children's bodies

There has been a particular focus on children and the problem of 'childhood obesity' in the medical, public health and health policy literature and in the popular media since the beginning of the 'obesity epidemic' discourse. Claims have been made that levels of overweight and obesity in children in western countries have risen dramatically since the late 1990s, and that their current and future health will be adversely affected as a result. Thus, for example, a two-page newspaper article focusing on childhood obesity published in a Sydney newspaper in November 2011 made the now well-rehearsed claims that 'Childhood obesity has become an epidemic … Almost a quarter of Australian children are overweight or obese and doctors fear that if the trend continues this generation of children will die younger than their parents' (Browne 2011: 8).

Several writers from the sociology of education and children's geography have focused their attentions on the ways in which children's bodies are regulated and governed via the discourses and strategies associated with concerns about body weight. Some of these scholars use the term 'biopedagogical' strategies or alternatively 'body pedagogies' to refer to the ways in which individuals are taught or trained to view and use their bodies in specific ways via education. For some commentators from this perspective, governmental strategies and anti-obesity policies directed at children and young people goes beyond concerns about members of this target group's weight and health to attempts to regulate and manage them in general. They assert that the 'obesity crisis' discourse allows and condones the intervention of surveillance strategies into increasingly wider dimensions of children and young people's everyday lives (Gard and Wright 2005; Evans *et al.* 2008; Colls and Evans 2009; Harwood 2009; Rich and Evans 2009).

These writers have pointed out that whereas in previous eras schools were encouraged to teach students about physical fitness and healthy eating practices as part of an overall focus on good health, the emergence of 'obesity epidemic' discourse has resulted in such efforts being reframed as predominantly about weight control. As a result, children have become a specific target for state-sponsored anti-obesity strategies, as evinced by the American 'Let's Move' campaign and Taskforce on Childhood Obesity and the British 'Change4Life' campaign. Given that it is possible to monitor large numbers of children in educational settings, schools are seen as the ideal sites for educating children and young people about what have been identified in the biomedical literature as the causes of fatness and developing programmes of physical activity and dietary practices believed to alleviate the health risks of fatness. Technologies of measurement and surveillance directed at students' weight control have also been increasingly employed in schools, including fingerprint screening to monitor students' lunch choices, regular weighing and height measurements to calculate BMI, the use of pedometers to count how many steps young people take throughout the day, skinfold measurements and lunch box inspections. Here again, virtual and abstracted governmental assemblages are created which are divorced from the lived embodied realities of young people's daily lives (Evans and Colls 2009; Rich and Evans 2009; Rich et al. 2011).

These strategies and policies of surveillance and measurement and the creation of governmental assemblages focused on obesity potentially have negative repercussions for the young people they target. Many critics in the social sciences have expressed their concern about the messages that children and young people may be receiving about body size in relation to obesity prevention education. They claim that a focus on body weight may exacerbate the low self-esteem that many young people may feel in relation to their appearance, particularly those who are overweight or obese, or encourage eating disorders such as anorexia and bulimia. So too, they are concerned that increasing a focus on school-based physical activity may prove counterproductive by forcing students into such activity for the sake of reducing their body weight. This may particularly be the case for those children identified as overweight or obese who are then subjected to special attention and monitoring and sometimes required to perform additional physical exercise, dubbed 'fat laps' in some schools. Fat children, therefore, are singled out and stigmatized, in some cases publicly shamed, and all children are encouraged to see physical exercise as a means to lose weight rather than as an activity enjoyed for its own sake (Gard and Wright 2005; Evans et al. 2008; Beausoleil 2009; Rail 2009; Rich and Evans 2009; Rich et al. 2011).

Some writers use the term 'disordered eating' to encompass not only over-eating but also unhealthy eating, continual attempts at dieting, extreme weight-control measures, binge eating and at the more extreme, anorexia and bulimia, and argue that these behaviours may affect students who have been influenced by the extreme focus on controlling body weight in schools (Evans *et al.* 2008; Beausoleil 2009). It has been argued that for middle-class girls, in particular, the emphasis in schools generally on high performance, expectations of doing well academically, requires of students an intense degree of self-control and hard work. This focus on performance also conforms to the prevailing focus in education on regulating and disciplining the body to prevent weight gain. It serves to engender feelings of stress in the quest to achieve these ideals of perfection. Many such girls subsequently develop feelings of guilt, shame and self-doubt and a need to take control over their bodies that culminates in some in the development of disordered eating problems. While, therefore, the intense emphasis in schools on performance and achievement does not in itself cause disordered eating, it may potentially contribute to the conditions in which these problems are generated (Evans *et al.* 2008).

The family as site of intervention

The family setting has also provided an integral site for governmental interventions into children and young people's weight control. Health policy documents and health promotional material have regularly positioned parents, and specifically, mothers, as primarily responsible for monitoring and regulating their children's body weight (Burrows 2009; Fullagar 2009; Evans *et al.* 2011). The popular media have similarly placed great emphasis on parental responsibility for their children's body weight, including such television programmes as *Honey We're Killing the Kids* and *Jamie Oliver's Food Revolution* (see also Chapter 4). Many such appeals focus on parents' desire to be able to engage in active leisure pursuits with their children or live long enough to see them grow up. Parents are urged to provide a 'good example' to their children by engaging in the recommended weight-control practices themselves, and to keep a close eye on their children's weight, dietary intake and exercise habits (Burrows 2009; Fullagar 2009).

This focus on mothers' responsibility for their children's weight begins in pregnancy, when women deemed overweight or obese are advised to lose weight for the benefit of their foetus, to the point that they are discursively positioned as posing a risk to their foetuses if they fail to lose weight (Boero 2009; Keenan and Stapleton 2010; McNaughton 2011). Once the child is born, mothers are then charged with the responsibility of ensuring that their children do not become fat and that they themselves act as good 'role models' by engaging in practices of the self which are recommended to avoid becoming overweight. If their children are deemed overweight, then it is assumed that their mothers are to blame, to the point that accusations of 'child abuse' have been levelled at mothers of extremely obese children and threats made to remove them from their families (Bell *et al.* 2009; McNaughton 2011). Popular media discourses have continually referred to children being neglected by their mothers by being allowed to eat too much 'junk food' or watch too much television (Boero 2009; Rich and Evans 2009). As a result, many mothers position themselves as primarily responsible for their children's diet and body weight and evince feelings of guilt and shame if they feel that they have not conformed sufficiently to these imperatives (Fullagar 2009).

This idealized figure assumes a concept of 'good motherhood' which demands constant surveillance of oneself (as a role model) and one's children to ward off the threat of obesity, and requires women to simultaneously supply and deny food to their children. Maternal love is directly linked to feeding children with food that is officially deemed healthy, and those mothers who are perceived to have 'failed' to protect their children from fatness are portrayed as irresponsible. Mothers who are viewed as allowing their children to over-eat or eat the wrong kinds of foods are portrayed as permissive and over-indulgent, incapable of properly disciplining their children's eating habits by saying 'no'. Fat children are represented in this discourse as out-of-control and their mothers as weak and ineffectual (Bell *et al.* 2009; Boero 2009; Halse 2009).

Thus, for example, many of the television advertisements for the 'Change4Life' campaign specifically addressed mothers as the providers of food for the family, particularly working-class mothers, who in the policy documentation of the campaign were positioned as requiring more assistance to provide appropriate food for their families. The background documentation represented mothers' love for their children as sometimes resulting in misguided, irrational and overly indulging attempts to give them unhealthy foods or too much food, as did television advertisements which referred to mothers over-feeding their children. Excessive or inappropriate affective relations between mothers and their children, in which mothers failed to take responsibility and to exert authority over their children, were thus directly linked to fatness in the children. The campaign attempted instead to substitute affective with 'rational' judgements on the part of mothers. 'Really loving' one's child was portrayed as giving them the 'right' food and preventing them from becoming obese, even if it meant constant battles with children who wanted other foods (Evans *et al.* 2011).

Minority groups and weight control

Other groups singled out for attention in official discourses on obesity include members of the working class, the poor and those from minority ethnic or racial groups. Like women, members of these marginalized and socially and economically disadvantaged groups tend to be represented as lacking the self-discipline required to achieve and maintain a thin body. The idealized contained and controlled thin body is not only male, but also white and middle class. Other bodies are compared and contrasted against this ideal, and often found lacking. So too, cultural aspects such as traditional ethnic diets are represented as inferior to that of the middle-class white diet and stigmatized for their differences (Kirkland 2011). The focus on measurement technologies in the school setting, for example, not only positions white fat children as Other, but also non-white children, who are often disproportionally represented among those identified as overweight or obese (Azzarito 2009; Burrows 2009). In the family context, mothers of non-white ethnic or racial groups are positioned as particularly neglectful in allowing their children to become fat, and it is assumed that such mothers require special 'education' so that they can more effectively perform their responsibilities in monitoring their children's weight (Bell *et al.* 2009; Boero 2009; Evans *et al.* 2011; McNaughton 2011).

This linking of non-white ethnicity or race, and the poor and working class with the inability to regulate embodiment and control body weight goes back to the nineteenth century, in which notions of racial and class superiority shaped views on health and illness (Lupton 1995; Petersen and Lupton 1996). In the United States, attempts to contain the 'contamination' of immigrants and newly emancipated black Americans by utilizing concepts of 'hygiene' and eugenics shaped hierarchies of classes of social groups. A predisposition to fatness was viewed as part of the inherited traits of the 'lower classes' and non-white or Jewish immigrants who were positioned as 'inferior' and 'primitive' compared to the 'superior' and 'civilized' middle-class and upper-middle-class white Americans. By the early twentieth century, the slim body was positioned as the most civilized type, as it represented the privileged cultural values of self-restraint and self-control which members of 'primitive' social groups were seen to lack (Farrell 2009; Gilman 2010).

Discourses on overweight and obesity tend to homogenize racial and ethnic groups, assuming that they are all the same in their behaviour and genetic makeup. Members of minority ethnic and racial groups are constantly represented as less physically active, based on cultural stereotypes and assumptions, while working class or poor people are assumed to be ignorant due to poor education levels and to require additional resources to educate them about appropriate behaviours for weight control. Little awareness is demonstrated in dominant discursive representations of people from non-white or economically disadvantaged groups that such individuals' own understandings and beliefs concerning food consumption, fitness, fatness and the ideal body may value aspects which differ from those of mainstream official obesity science and policy (Azzarito 2009; Burrows 2009; Kirkland 2011). Thus, for example, interviews with both black and white Canadians found that black women were far more likely than white women and all men to express resistance towards obesity discourse and the notions that thinness is equivalent to healthiness and that the BMI was an accurate measurement of healthy body weight (Ristovski-Slijepcevic et al. 2010).

4

THE TRANSGRESSIVE FAT BODY

Why does the fat body inspire such visceral and negative emotional responses? Why is it subject to such rigid attempts to control and contain it? This chapter addresses these questions by examining the concepts of transgression, the abject and the grotesque body and the ways in which the binary opposition between Self and Other is maintained via the projection of feelings of disgust and revulsion upon the fat body.

Fatness and morality

The appearance and deportment of the body conveys specific cultural meanings to those who observe this body. Certain features of bodily appearance are 'read' or interpreted by oneself and others as denoting aspects of the individual within that body. By virtue of the sociocultural meanings that are attached to these bodily features, various assumptions are made about the self which are inextricably part of that body (Grosz 1995). Many of these assumptions adhere to dominant binary oppositions, such as male/female, white/black, civilized/wild, contained/ grotesque, normal/pathological and healthy/sick. The body thus confesses what are believed to be 'truths' about the inner self within this body. The sheer fleshly appearance of size of the fat body is thus itself a symbol that is read in various ways by those who view this body and those who inhabit it. Fat bodies take up more space than other bodies: they draw attention – the gaze of others – by virtue of their size. This gaze is often judgemental and moralizing in its interpretation of the flesh it surveys.

The constant association of fatness with disease and ill health results in the fat body bearing the negative meanings of illness. Illness and disease have long carried the symbolic meanings of loss of control, disorder and chaos and threatened rationality (Lupton 2012). To be ill in contemporary societies is already to be marginalized, because illness is treated as a bodily state which challenges expectations about the well-functioning, productive citizen. As noted in Chapter 3, in societies where good citizens manage, regulate and protect their health, to fail to do so, to become ill or die prematurely, is viewed as a failure of personal responsibility.

Ill people are continually subject to moralistic assumptions about their 'lifestyle choices', particularly if they overtly flout public health or medical advice. When an illness is viewed as resulting from carelessness, lack of self-discipline or licentious or illegal behaviour, the ill person becomes treated with moral opprobrium (see the essays in Brandt and Rozin 1997a; Lupton 1994, 1995, 2012).

Obesity shares aspects of the moralizing discourses which give meaning to many medical conditions which are believed to be the result of 'lifestyle choices', such as lung conditions caused by smoking, liver conditions caused by excessive alcohol consumption, hepatitis spread through injecting drug use or sexually transmissible diseases. Indeed, there are many similarities between the cultural representation of obesity and those portraying HIV/AIDS, particularly when the latter condition emerged in the 1980s. In both cases, certain bodily practices – male-to-male sexual practices, promiscuous heterosexuality or injecting drug use in the case of HIV/AIDS, and in the case of fat people, over-eating and laziness – were identified as causing disease. Gay men, heterosexuals with many partners and injecting drug users were stigmatized and singled out in the news media as deviant in their bodily practices, as lacking the requisite self-control to prevent HIV infection, just as fat people have been the subject of discourses concerning their deviant and uncontrolled physical practices, their tendency to give in to intemperate desires (Lupton 1994; Brandt and Rozin 1997b).

The moral meanings associated with fat embodiment not only draw upon contemporary medical discourses, but have long antecedents in religious ideas about the body. It is only very recently that dietary control and body size have been pre-dominantly considered as a health problem. Instead there is a strong historical link between concepts of the body and food consumption with religious and spiritual beliefs. The ancient Greeks saw the control of body weight as part of the spiritual relationship between food, the body and the gods. Fatness in both ancient Greek and Roman medical thought and practice was seen as a pathological result of bodily imbalance (Gilman 2010).

The emergence of Christianity intensified the link between holiness, spirituality, asceticism and a thin body shape. Judeo-Christian ethics developed a belief system around the practices of eating and fasting as holy rituals, which themselves are built upon concepts of health and spirituality developed by the ancients. The early Christians represented the body as God's temple, and thus the fat and unhealthy body was a sign of a faulty relationship with God, moral corruptness and an opening of the body to sin via gluttony. Gluttony was linked to sexual appetite and viewed both as animalistic and evidence of a body out-of-control. To deprive oneself of food was considered as the ultimate test of self-discipline. The pious body was gaunt and emaciated, demonstrating control of fleshly desires, while the fat body was the embodiment of sin and the inability to discipline one's desires. Early Christian writers commented upon their struggles with indulging their desire for food and drink. Taking pleasure in eating for satisfaction rather than simply fuelling the body was considered giving in to the sins of the flesh (Bynum 1987; Klein 2001; Gilman 2010).

The 'science of diet' and the concept of the 'body as machine' developing in the nineteenth century began to delineate which types of foods should be eaten, and in what quantities, to avoid a fat body. Discourses on fatness become less overtly linked to Christian beliefs and more overtly to the pronouncements of 'science'. However moral assumptions based on religious beliefs were still made about the link between fatness and self-indulgence. The development of psychology resulted in a view on fatness, for example, which positioned it as a weakness of the will. These new ideas about health and body functioning drew on long-established beliefs about the importance of controlling the body's consumption as a moral and ethical enterprise. Indeed religion appropriated the arguments of the new science to provide rationales for obesity, to the point where, in the contemporary era, science and morality based on Christian tenets continue to work together to give meaning to fatness and the fat subject (Turner 1991; Lupton 1996; Gilman 2010).

Fat bodies in the popular media

I referred in Chapter 1 to *The Biggest Loser*, a reality television series which first screened in the United States in 2004 but which then was produced in local versions in many countries, including the United Kingdom, Australia, various European and Asian countries, South Africa, Brunei and other Arabic countries (Anonymous 2012). I noted the extreme humiliation and shame to which contestants on that programme were subjected, including public displays of their fat bodies and weigh-ins in which their body weights were displayed on giant screens.

Television programmes such as *The Biggest Loser* and other reality series centred on weight loss and lifestyle behaviours such as the programmes *Honey, We're Killing the Kids* and *Jamie Oliver's Fast Food Revolution* achieve high ratings, demonstrating an intense level of interest from the television-watching public. The popular media in the early decades of the twenty-first century and their consumers are obsessed not only with such displays of weight loss from 'ordinary' people, but also with the size, shape and relative adiposity of celebrities' bodies. Popular magazines, television programmes and websites focused on celebrities' lives routinely celebrate and congratulate celebrities (nearly all of whom are female) on their weight loss if they appear to have slimmed down. Conversely, these celebrities are regularly castigated and ridiculed if they appear to have put on weight. Their bodies are shown in detail in visual images which home in on any sign of abdominal bulging or cellulite. Women such as the Kardashian sisters, Kelly Osbourne, Tyra Banks, Oprah Winfrey, Britney Spears and Kirstie Allen, all of whose weight appears to change dramatically from plump or overweight to acceptably slim and back again, are constantly subjected to surveillance and judgement in these forums.

Indeed, there are a number of websites devoted to the portrayal of 'fat celebrities', showing 'before and after' photographs as their bodies morph from slim to fat. One website page, entitled '21 Celebrities That Got Fat' (Anonymous 2010) is particularly explicit in its judgemental and derisory tone, noting that 'Here are 21 celebrities that got beat down [sic] by the ugly stick'. Accompanying 'before and after' photographs provide a juxtaposition of sexually attractive and 'ugly' bodies, both male and female. While many of the celebrities featured still look attractive and well-groomed in the 'after' photographs, they are deemed 'ugly' simply because they have gained weight. There are also websites devoted to celebrities who are deemed to have gone 'too far' in weight loss, and now look very thin or almost emaciated, and it is suggested that they may be suffering from an eating disorder. The main emphasis remains on celebrities maintaining an appropriate slender physique, as long as they do not become 'scary skinny': a difficult balance for many to maintain in the continual glare of the spotlight.

Ordinary people's fat bodies are frequently portrayed in news media reporting of the 'obesity epidemic' as bulging and distended, often using close-up camera effects to distort their bodies beyond the reality of their fleshiness. Strategies of exposure and shaming are frequently used when representing fat bodies in news media and reality television programmes. Fat people are also often shown as gorging themselves with food, invariably food deemed to be 'unhealthy', such as hamburgers or chips. This visual link perpetuates the assumption that fatness is caused by the excessive and greedy consumption of the 'wrong' kinds of foods. A study of Australian news coverage of obesity, for example, noted recurring use of such derogatory expressions as 'fat arses', 'flabby flesh', 'lazy', 'unsightly slobs' and 'nuzzle their snouts into the trough' to describe fat people (Holland *et al.* 2011: 39). Combined with words often used in these reports such as 'bulging', 'flabby', 'getting fatter by the minute', the meanings conveyed are of alarming growth of the body to monstrous proportions (Lupton 1996; Inthorn and Boyce 2010; Holland *et al.* 2011).

Cooper (2007) has used the term 'headless fatties' to describe the common phenomenon in such media representations of fat people with their heads cropped off. Although presumably this technique is employed by the media organizations to preserve people's privacy by not showing their faces, the consequence of such visual portrayals is that fat bodies are depersonalized and objectified. They are transformed from people with individual identities to lumps of flesh, there to provide a vivid literal lesson of what can happen if people 'allow' themselves to become fat.

Programmes such as *Honey, We're Killing the Kids* and *Jamie Oliver's Fast Food Revolution*, as well as Oliver's earlier series

Jamie's Ministry of Food, focus on families with young children. In these series there is much agonized discussion about fat children and about how their parents are 'killing' them by 'allowing' them to become fat. The presenters convey a sympathetic tone to the parents when advising them how to ensure that their children will live to adulthood free of disabling health conditions that allegedly will be caused by the children's fatness, with an 'I am here to help' presentation of the expert self. Nonetheless, they attempt to provoke guilt, fear and shame in the parents by the ways in which their children's body size and dietary and exercise habits are described. For example, as part of this regime of expert advice directed at frightening parents into changing their parenting habits, they are confronted with computer-generated images of what (supposedly) their children will look like as adults if they continue with their lifestyle habits. Invariably the children are presented in these images as fat, unattractive and unhealthy-looking. There is much emphasis, therefore, on physical appearance and the representation of the future fat adult's body as gross, repugnant and ill, a body to be avoided at all costs.

The grotesque fat body

The images described above conform to a long-standing discourse on fat embodiment which represents it as grotesque. Grotesque bodies deviate from the norm, mainly by exceeding it. They defy clear definitions and borders and occupy the liminal middle ground between life and death. They are permeable and uncontained, transgressive of their own limits. They are the embodiment of ambiguity, which in itself creates apprehension in a cultural context in which ambiguity challenges privileged notions of certainty. Grotesque bodies are, above all, carnal: that is, they are overtly fleshly and expressive of desire rather than the simply neutral containers for the disembodied consciousness which is such a valued ideal of the body in western culture (Bakhtin 1965; Shabot 2006).

The grotesque fat body stands in a binary opposition of symbolic meaning against the civilized thin body. The former body is portrayed as uncontained, uncontrolled, permeable and open to the world, while the latter is represented as tightly contained, closed off from the world. Fatness and thinness are part of this meaning system associated with the importance of control and containment of the body/self. Given the dominant cultural model of the 'body as machine', in which it is understood that energy taken in and used has a direct relationship with body mass (Gard and Wright 2005), in concert with the Cartesian concept of the body as separated from, and ruled by the mind, it is assumed that the thin body represents the ability to rigidly control one's food intake. In contrast, fat bodies, which themselves are portrayed as excessive in their fleshly abundance, are regarded as the physical manifestation of their owners' lack of self-control and self-discipline, their tendency to over-consume and lack the self-discipline to keep their food intake moderate and exercise appropriately. Excess desire, in this logic, is represented by excess flesh.

People who allow themselves to become fat are described as 'letting themselves go': that is, as relinquishing control over their bodies, loosening the restraints of self-discipline (Hartley 2001). Fat flesh, therefore, is viewed as not only repugnant in its physical manifestation of bodily excess and lack of containment, but also as denoting the self's inferiority. The common notion that 'inside every fat person there is a thin person trying to get out' implies that fat flesh imprisons the 'authentic' subject within. Fat flesh is viewed as inauthentic, a kind of disguise for the real self. Fat bodies are Other to the privileged contained and disciplined Self. Even fat people may constitute their corpulent flesh as Other to their 'real self', while thin people regard fat people as the Other they strenuously seek to avoid becoming.

Fatness, disgust, abjection

Concepts of loathing, revulsion and disgust are redolent in contemporary western cultures' representations of the fat bodies (Shapiro 1994; Hartley 2001; Kent 2001; Murray 2008). Fat flesh challenges notions of propriety because of its fluidity and excessiveness. It is wobbly and jiggly, it hangs loosely, it oozes over into over people's spaces, confronts them with its monstrous dimensions. Hence the oft-referred to figure of the fat person who takes up too much space in the tight confines of the aeroplane seat, whose flesh intrudes from its 'proper' place into one's own space, evoking annoyance or even anger, but also contempt and revulsion at its lack of containment and therefore propriety.

Murray's (2008: 11) vivid account of her perceptions of her own fat embodiment as she sits in a doctor's surgery emphasizes the sheer fluidity of fat flesh:

> In the doctor's eyes I become vast and amorphous. Under his gaze, I feel myself ooze over the sides of the chair, my flesh drooping, dripping down the chair legs, pooling oleaginous on the floor before them ... I seem to spread and spread in the room, filling the corners of the office with my fat flesh ... I am a fleshy ooze.

Murray's words convey both the grotesque nature of her fat flesh and her own disgust for it as she imagines how the doctor must perceive her. By her own admission her grotesque body is contaminating, soiling and revolting in its lack of containment, its oiliness and propensity to spread over boundaries. These words are redolent of the self-hatred which fat people may feel towards their own bodies as well as their perceptions of how others see them.

Disgust is also evident the reaction towards other people's fat bodies quoted below:

> My body feels a revulsion to their heaviness, largeness, looseness. I watch in disgust as they manoeuvre, calculating aisle widths, chair size, furniture strengths. Folds of flesh hang from chins, arms and bellies. I feel the weight of the loose, fat filled skin. A churning in my stomach and the rising of a bile taste in my throat is my visceral response to the sight of them.
>
> *(Shapiro 1994: 71)*

Disgust is often used in educational strategies in the classroom, media reports and public health campaigns to elicit concern about oneself becoming fat (Leahy 2009). Disgust is associated with moral meaning: it is evoked by the sense that 'something is wrong' and that this anomaly must be put to rights. This emotional response to fatness combines, therefore, a sensory reaction to the sight of bodily excess with moral opprobrium about how the body came to grow so large and uncontained.

The concept of abjection addresses the subconscious level of the reaction of disgust. For Kristeva (1982), the abject is that which is difficult to contain, which is liminal and crosses bodily boundaries. Its lack of definition and its liminal status inspire feelings of revulsion and fear of contamination. The abject is an external menace, something from which we must protect ourselves, but there is also a sense that it is somehow contained within us, and must be expelled from oneself to achieve integrity of the body. Disgust is generated by this dual response to the external and internal threat, to the idea that the abject might be contained within the self.

The uncontained nature of the fat body, its looseness and liquidity, its lack of defined boundaries and tendency to ooze, inspires abjection. The abject fat body inspires a desire to distance oneself from it and also to prevent one's own body becoming similarly abject. Attempts to reduce the size of the fat body via dieting, exercise, drugs or weight surgery, therefore, may be conceptualized as attempts to counter the abjection of the fat of the body within oneself, to expel it. When fatness is viewed on others' bodies, it represents this abject substance that is externalized and the fear and disgust we feel about our own potentially uncontained bodies are thus projected onto the Other's body. So too, because of the continual cultural linking of the fat body with death and disease, the fat body inspires fear and revulsion as it is perceived as a body already in the process of dying. The fat body serves as a site for the projection of fears about death and bodily decay, a means of maintaining boundaries of the 'good Self' (Kent 2001).

Femininities, fluidities, fatness

As I noted in Chapter 2, feminist scholars have been central in constructing critiques of the imperatives in contemporary western cultures for women, in particular, to be slender. For at least four decades, since the emergence of second-wave feminism, feminist critics have pointed out that notions of what type and size of body constitutes an ideal, attractive female body underpin the valuing of thinness and the stigmatizing of fatness for women. Susie Orbach's (1978) book *Fat is a Feminist Issue* was an influential, ground-breaking work in drawing attention to body size issues for women from an overtly feminist perspective. Many books and journal articles since then have been published by feminist scholars on the topic of body weight and the feminine body.

In the 1980s and 1990s there was a distinct focus in the feminist literature on the eating disorders anorexia and bulimia. Many feminist critics argued that the intense pressures on girls and women to achieve and maintain the idealized thin female body resulted in the majority of women keeping themselves on a perpetual diet and weighing themselves continually, with some succumbing to debilitating eating disorders. While such works did investigate the meanings of fatness in the context of the thin ideal, their predominant focus was on the 'average' woman or girl who mistakenly viewed herself as fat and thus devoted much time and emotional energy to dieting and exercising to achieve a thinner body. Reference was commonly made in such works to the 'cult' or the 'tyranny' of thinness and how this idealized slender body affected most women's lives because they could never feel as though they could achieve this ideal. Mass media representations of the female fat body were a particular focus of feminist critics, who showed persuasively how images of fashion models and celebrities, and images and discourses in advertising constantly presented thin women as the attractive ideal and fat women as repugnant and asexual (see, for example, Chernin 1981; Bordo 1993; Hesse-Biber 1996). Since the early 2000s, with the emergence of the 'obesity epidemic', the attention of feminist writers interested in women and body weight issues has largely shifted to the dilemmas of fat embodiment and there is now a substantial feminist literature on this topic.

Feminist scholars have contended that female embodiment has been considered problematic in western cultures because of the symbolic meanings of disorder, lack of containment and inability to control body boundaries that have traditionally been associated with women's bodies. Women's bodies are conceptualized as permeable, leaky, more open to the world by virtue of their supposed volatile emotionality and their particularly female body processes such as menstruation, lactation, pregnancy, birth and menopause, all of which involve the uncontrolled exiting of bodily fluids from their bodies. The bodily states of pregnancy and childbirth also challenge notions of Self/Other, of the containment of the subject, in their blurring of the boundaries between one's own body and that of another body (Kristeva 1982; Bordo 1993; Grosz 1994; Shildrick 1997; Longhurst 2001). Cultural responses to fat female bodies draw upon these already well-established ideas about the uncontained, uncontrolled female body.

It has been contended that the supposed emotionality of women, their tendency to express their emotions more openly and feel them more strongly, is also closely linked to the stereo-typical concept of the fat woman. Fat women are regarded as particularly emotionally volatile, using eating as an emotional escape, compulsively eating without being able to control their consumption (Murray 2008). Just like the bulimic woman, the fat woman is regarded as someone bearing emotional problems which manifest in a tendency to gorge herself with food. The bulimic then vomits out the food, and remains thin or 'normal' in her weight: the fat woman keeps it inside and remains fat.

The size of the fat female body also challenges cultural expectations. Women have been encouraged in contemporary western societies to take up as little space as possible, to contain their bodies by keeping their arms and legs close to the body and not allowing their flesh to grow too large. Largeness of the body is seen as unfeminine, as a male attribute: women are expected to look dainty, weak and fragile, as part of their subordination to men. Some feminists argue, indeed, that the growing influence of women in the public sphere, in high-achieving professional occupations, has been accompanied by the increasing focus on women keeping their bodies small, because of the threat they pose to masculine power (Hartley 2001; Longhurst 2001). By virtue of its size, the female fat body is simultaneously asexual and hypersexual. Female fat bodies demonstrate large and prominent breasts, hips and buttocks, all sexually coded as particular signs of feminine embodiment. However, because fat women are viewed as more masculine, as ugly and unfeminine, they are rendered culturally asexual, as it is assumed that no man would desire them (Hartley 2001; Longhurst 2001, 2005; Murray 2008). Indeed interviews with fat women have found that some feel less feminine because of their large body size and are often treated by men as asexual for the same reason (Tischner and Malson 2011; Gailey 2012).

Interestingly, anorexic bodies and fat bodies are understood and represented in popular culture in similar ways. Both are highly feminized, viewed in the case of anorexics as the result of neurotic and over-controlled femininity, and for fat women out-of-control feminine urges. Both are viewed as asexual, because their bodies are so extreme in size that they do not conform to idealized notions of female beauty. Both are portrayed as spectacles, freakish and abnormal. Both are viewed as emotionally damaged, either choosing to avoid eating for emotionally disturbed reasons, or eating too much to fulfil emotional needs. Both are viewed as irrational in their desires and thought-processes and failing to see that through their choices around food and exercise they are slowly killing themselves: the anorexic by starvation, the fat woman by making herself ever fatter. For both, food becomes a material object invested with tremendous power, able to entice the individual to lose control over herself. The bodies of both are subject to a high degree of monitoring and surveillance. For both anorexics and fat women, their body size is an integral part of their identity. So too, some anorexics and fat women reject medicalized discourses on their bodies, which represent them as pathological, for a view which defines their bodies as 'normal'.

Spoilt masculinities and fat embodiment

Due to the fact that most critiques of the cultural dimensions of fat embodiment have emerged from feminist scholars, the focus has been on women and their experience of fatness. Yet the smaller literature on fat men has demonstrated that they experience similar feelings of shame, humiliation and revulsion about their bodies and are also treated by others as inferior, deficient and lacking in self-control (Gill 2008; Brandon and Pritchard 2011; Monaghan and Hardey 2011). The preoccupation with dieting and controlling body weight which has been evident in western societies for more than a century has included men as well as women in its purview. Indeed most of the early proponents of body weight control were men writing about their own theories and experiences, as were their followers

(Turner 1991; Bell and McNaughton 2007; Gilman 2010; Monaghan and Hardey 2011).

Fat embodiment in a man in some ways poses a strong challenge to hegemonic ideals of masculinity. While thinness may not be a central dimension of the ideal male body as it is represented in popular culture, strength, physical fitness and highly developed muscularity are idealized, while flabbiness, loose flesh and paunches are reviled (Bell and McNaughton 2007). The 'six-pack' stomach and well-muscled chest is the ultimate symbol of the sought-after male body, while the pregnant-like 'beer belly' and flaccid, fleshy, female-like chest (sometimes derisively described as 'man boobs') stand as its despised opposite. As noted above, ideal masculine bodies are expected to be tightly contained, their body boundaries rigidly kept closed from the outside world. In sharp contrast, male fat bodies are portrayed as soft, flabby, lacking the muscularity and strength of the 'normal' idealized male body. They are therefore considered as far closer to the stereotypical feminine body in their softness, roundness and fleshiness. So too, as noted above, fatness itself tends to be associated with excessive femininity.

Given the continual coding of fatness as feminine, a property of particularly unregulated and uncontained female embodiment, fat men are viewed as effeminate rather than masculine in their soft roundness and lack of apparent virility. Their bodies lack the phallic hardness of the idealized male body, and thus the fat man is expected to lack sexual desire or attractiveness to women. Dominant cultural representations of the fat man constantly present him as a childlike, bumbling oaf, lacking typical masculine authority and power (Mosher 2001). Homer Simpson is the archetypal fat man on television: soft and round-bodied, stupid, greedy, lazy, worthy only of contempt.

The Northern English men interviewed by Monaghan (Monaghan 2007; Monaghan and Hardey 2011) used the term 'fat bastard' to describe themselves and others considered fat. While this term sometimes suggests a sense of masculine pride about being fat, it is also often used in a pejorative sense, to denote lack of self-control and physical unattractiveness. The 'proud fat bastard', in some websites referred to as the 'Big Handsome Man' (see Monaghan 2005b, and also Chapter 6), defines his fatness as part of his enjoyment in the sensual pleasures of life, such as pub culture or the gluttonous enjoyment of food, or alternatively as a nonchalance or contempt about placing importance on one's physical health. The working-class self-defined 'fat bastard' positions himself as resisting the constricting expectations of medical and public health discourses about body weight, and middle-class sensibilities about the importance of maintaining strict control over one's body to achieve a particular body aesthetic. Nonetheless, some ambivalence is also evident among such men. Claiming the 'fat bastard' label to describe oneself is sometimes employed as part of a preemptive strike against others deriding one's body size. Some of the men interviewed by Monaghan certainly exhibited signs of identifying with the 'spoiled identity' referred to by Goffman (1963) as part of their self-labelling as 'fat bastards' (see also Gill 2008). The 'fat bastard' moniker, therefore, both reflects and resists the pejorative meanings of the fat male body, depending on who uses it and in what context.

Despite the disgust and contempt levelled at fat men's bodies, men themselves may find it difficult to engage in weight-reduction activities such as dieting because of the feminine coding of such activities and their linking to body consciousness, vanity and obsession with one's appearance, all of which are considered negatively and as stereotypically feminine (or homosexual) and narcissistic concerns (Gill 2008; Mallyon *et al.* 2010). Even to appear to be concerned about one's physical appearance and to want to take steps to do something to change it is derided in normative male culture as 'girly' or 'gay'. Australian men who were participating in a diet trial, for example, were reluctant to let others know that they were dieting in the attempt to reduce weight as this posed a threat to their sense of masculinity

(Mallyon *et al.* 2010). So too, interviews with men in various parts of England and Australia found that while they articulated and valued the idea of 'taking care' of one's body by engaging in weight control practices and expressed very negative attitudes towards becoming overweight, they also expressed the idea that becoming too obsessive or narcissistic about this was inappropriate for a man (Gill 2008).

A study of male members of a slimming club located in Northern England found that they tended to employ 'muscle talk' to explain some of the excess size and weight of their bodies. The men claimed that because they had developed larger muscles, this accounted for a heavier weight. These men were concerned about losing too much weight, resulting in a body that looked emaciated or gaunt. They remarked that such a body looked ill rather than healthy. Carrying some extra weight was valued over being too thin, given that male bodies were expected to be large rather than slight. Such research demonstrates the contingency of how 'fatness' or 'obesity' is defined. Some of the men who had lost a great deal of weight no longer saw themselves as fat and were happy with their weight, despite the fact that they were still defined as overweight or obese according to their BMI. These men were able to challenge the concept that the BMI should be the sole means of defining obesity (Monaghan 2007).

While there is a plethora of interesting and insightful work in the humanities and social sciences on the fluidities and porosity of women's bodies, some of which is discussed above, little has been published which analyses the meanings of men's bodily fluidities, with the important exception of work on HIV/AIDS and homosexuality. The messiness and leakiness of that category of body which is represented as ideally contained in comparison to all other bodies – that of the white, youthful, heterosexual, able-bodied male – has rarely been examined (Longhurst 2001). Longhurst's (2001) research with New Zealand and Scottish people in managerial work positions, both men and women, found that the interviewees strongly emphasized the importance of presenting a corporate body image at work. This involved being well-groomed, wearing the standard 'corporate uniform' of a business suit and having a body that was physically fit and not overweight. All these practices of the self combined to present a corporate identity that was considered tightly controlled of its body boundaries, impervious to outside penetration and therefore powerful and rational. 'Looking good' was a major part of presenting a successful managerial self for both men and women. The unfit, flabby, fat body was viewed as failing to achieve this ideal image. As one male manager put it, 'the fat slob in an expensive suit is still a fat slob in an expensive suit. It's not a nice thing to say but it's a reality' (quoted in Longhurst 2001: 114).

5

BEING/FEELING FAT

What does it feel like to be a fat person in a cultural context in which fat is reviled? How are fat bodies discriminated against, how do fat people feel about their bodies and their weight-loss efforts, what are their experiences of moving around in space and place? Should fatness be considered a disability? This chapter addresses these questions.

Fat discrimination

'Fat loathing', 'fat hatred', 'fat oppression', 'thin supremacies', 'fat phobia', 'a witch hunt targeting fatness and fat people', 'weight prejudice' – these terms and others have been commonly employed by fat activists to describe the stigma and judgemental reactions faced by fat people. Fat people are underprivileged and face stigmatization and prejudice in number of socioeconomic arenas. Compared with others, they are statistically more likely to live in poverty, earn less income, be unemployed, have lower education levels, be employed in lower status jobs and experience lower living standards. In social terms, fat people receive less respect from shop assistants, are less likely to be married and are often subjected to derogatory humour and pejorative comments from co-workers, friends and family members and in public settings from strangers. They are viewed negatively by healthcare providers, who often see them as lazy, stupid, non-compliant and worthless and judge their fatness as being caused by lack of will-power. Fat people often avoid attending medical appointments because of their concerns about being weighed and then judged negatively by the doctor. Fat children are subjected to greater harassment and prejudice than other children, and experience ostracism, teasing and bullying to a greater extent (Ernsberger 2009; Halse 2009; Wann 2009).

Whether or not socioeconomic disadvantage leads to fatness, or whether fatness itself causes poverty and other forms of social and economic disadvantage is a point of debate. The kinds of discrimination against fat people described above can result in them not being able to obtain more highly paid employment, for example. It has also been contended that the lower socio-economic status of fat people may cause health problems, in which a combination of living in poverty, experiencing stigma based on body weight and accompanying diminished social status causes continuing stress. In conjunction with poor living conditions and the lack of opportunity to exercise and consume a high-quality diet, this exposure to stress may result in illness and disease, which are not treated effectively because of lack of access to high quality medical care (Ernsberger 2009).

The stigma and social ostracism and discrimination incurred by fat embodiment is similar in many ways to that of having the 'wrong' sexual preference, ethnicity or race, skin colour or religion, or having a disability. One major difference between these attributes and that of fatness, however, is that fatness is viewed in normative culture as self-incurred, as a bodily feature that can be altered if only the fat person had enough self-control and self-discipline. It is often assumed, therefore, that fat people are deserving of the discrimination they suffer because they brought it upon themselves by allowing their bodies to become fat.

The comments which Julie Guthman, an academic at the University of California at Santa Cruz, received from students who took her course on the politics of obesity are evidence of the ways in which fat people are negatively viewed by others (Guthman 2009b). Despite the course focusing in detail on the sceptical position on the 'obesity epidemic', the social construction and political dimensions of obesity and on fat activist arguments about obesity discourse, Guthman found that many of the students still articulated the dominant orthodox views that fatness is a negative and pathological state to be avoided at all costs and was evidence of an inability to take responsibility for one's health and appearance. Several students expressed highly negative views of one of the guest speakers, a well-known fat activist and proudly out fat woman, concerning her attempts to teach them that fatness need not be considered negatively. One student commented that 'I saw her as a quitter because she gave up on getting leaner and instead chose to embrace her blubbery self ... I think deep down she would love to lose some weight' (Guthman 2009b: 1121).

Guthman explains these reactions as evidence of the power and pervasiveness of the discourses of neoliberalism (Chapter 3), which so strongly privilege the notion of free subjects who take control over their destinies and thus are responsible for the trajectories of their lives. Her students found it very difficult not to view others' bodies and their own outside these discourses. Despite their exposure through the course to alternative ways of thinking, they still wanted to champion the notion that one should exercise responsibility and exert discipline over one's body: if not in the interests of health, then at the least to ensure that one is sexually attractive and able to 'get a date'. Body size was still viewed by many of them as a matter of personal choice, 'will-power' in resisting the temptation of food and the desire to 'take control of your life' or 'improving yourself'. 'Being fat is a choice, not a damn excuse for those lacking self control', as another student wrote (Guthman 2009b: 1126). Similar views have been constantly articulated in news media reports of obesity in western countries (Lupton 2004; Boero 2007; Saguy and Almeling 2008; Holland *et al.* 2011) and in documentaries and reality television programmes featuring fat people attempting to lose weight (Inthorn and Boyce 2010).

Fatness and the commodified body

In the discourse of the commodified body, the values of physical attractiveness and self-discipline have become elided. The outward body is believed to demonstrate the inner worthiness of the self: hence the focus on improving one's appearance. Looking youthful, slim and attractive is viewed as part of the continuing project of the self, in which the body is viewed as malleable and unfinished, requiring constant maintenance and work (Bordo 1993; Shilling 1993; Featherstone 2010; Wegenstein and Ruck 2011). Indeed, some commentators have referred to the current approach to viewing and assessing one's body and those of others as 'the cosmetic gaze'. This gaze is configured via the dominant discourses of technologies, practices and expectations around the concept of 'improving the body' so that it looks as attractive as possible (Wegenstein and Ruck 2011). In this notion of the body, self-discipline is about devoting the time, effort and money required to achieve and maintain one's 'best self'. These efforts must be constantly kept up, for the body threatens to fall into the disorder of ageing, flabbiness and fatness unless maintenance strategies are routinely undertaken.

In what I have elsewhere termed the 'food/health/beauty triplex' (Lupton 1996), food becomes categorized by how slimming or fattening it is, how it contributes to or detracts from the ideal of the healthy, slim body. As a consequence, it is difficult for many people to think about the food they are choosing to eat without deliberating over its caloric value and how it might affect their health or appearance. Even those people who do not view themselves as particularly fat find themselves implicated in this constant struggle over food consumption, leading in some cases to anxiety, guilt, shame and self-disgust as they attempt to conform to normative standards of health, beauty and self-control (Lupton 1996; Jallinoja *et al.* 2010). People who do identify as fat or overweight often represent their efforts as a battle with overwhelming urges to indulge in food. They are highly aware of the moral failure that their fat bodies represent (Gill 2008; Gimlin 2008; Murray 2008; Webb 2009; Monaghan and Hardey 2011; Tischner and Malson 2011).

Details of these efforts are found in many blogs on weight loss. The quotations below give some examples from a survey of such blogs I conducted in January 2012. Many such bloggers describe their efforts to lose weight as an intense struggle of their will to be slim against their almost overwhelming desires to over-eat, or to 'binge' on food. As one woman who calls herself Token Fat Girl and describes herself as 'a binge-eater' says on her blog: 'I'm obese, and it's not because of moderate or "normal" eating. It never has been, obviously. I've been thinking about my weight since I was eight years old and dieting for so long that I've never really known what normal eating looks or feels like.' So too, 'Dietgirl' notes that: 'Food has never just been food for me – it's been an escape from the world, a comfort and a coping mechanism.'

These bloggers also often describe their feelings of unhappiness about the appearance of their bodies and justify their efforts to lose weight as a way of looking good as well as feeling good. 'Skinny Hollie' talks about how she would love to change the appearance of her body and is finding the process of weight loss to be too protracted: 'I can't wait for that moment to get here where I like looking in the mirror again. I have been feeling kind of down about my appearance.' Similarly a different blogger writes that when she realized that she had put on a lot of weight, she felt that she had lost control of her body and was compelled to hide her excess flesh: 'I was now going to the beach with my friends and covering up for another reason. I felt ashamed. I felt ugly. I felt like some sort of animal.' She goes on to note that after losing quite a lot of weight 'I can also finally say I am happy with who I am and proud of what I have accomplished and overcome. Watch this space; I'm a work in progress.'

As these words suggest, even though many people no longer subscribe to the Judeo-Christian ethic of self-denial in pursuit of spirituality (discussed in Chapter 4), the expectation remains that asceticism is rewarded, if not with holiness, then with health and a sexually attractive appearance. Contemporary ideas about fat embodiment combine these older notions of morality and ethical deportment of the body, valuing the ability to resist the temptations of the flesh, with an aestheticized concept of the body. Maintaining a thin body is not only about disciplining desire but also achieving an appearance which conforms to normative ideals of beauty.

Fat people often find themselves constantly dieting, losing weight and then gaining it again, to the extent that some may actually choose to undergo bariatric (weight loss) surgery to end this constant battle over weight control (Throsby 2008, 2012; Murray 2009b). Some people who have undergone this procedure have viewed it as a way of normalizing their bodies to the extent that they are now able to gain some degree of control over their weight, seen as a 'first step' towards being able to engage in successful self-discipline. Rather than being 'controlled by food', such individuals are able to position themselves as exercising control, by virtue of the limits imposed on their food consumption and appetite by their post-surgical bodies. Interestingly, people who have lost weight due to a bariatric surgical procedure are often represented by themselves or others as having 'cheated'. Because the weight loss was caused by surgery, the moral high ground that otherwise these formerly fat people may have occupied by losing a great deal of weight is lost, because they have not done so by engaging in disciplined ascetic practices of the self (Throsby 2008).

Space, place and fat bodies

All bodies move and are visualized in spatial dimensions. Bodily experience and subjectivity are constructed through space and place in a dynamic and heterogeneous relationship with the physical world (Longhurst 2001). The interaction of bodies with other bodies, space and material objects produces a particular bodily assemblage, which may or may not find itself comfortably conforming to the dimensions offered by these spaces. Bodies which do not conform to the norm – because they are too small, too tall, too large, have disabilities, are too old or too young – may find that movement through, and fitting into, space becomes problematic. Rather than space and material objects being neutral and benign in their cultural meanings, therefore, they may be viewed as material and discursive constructions which contribute to the assemblage and disciplining of bodies (Longhurst 2001, 2005; Hetrick and Attig 2009).

Fat people are continually faced with the problem of fitting into space. The spatial dimensions of fatness include the difficulties of a larger body fitting within spaces meant for smaller bodies, such as seats on public transport, cinemas and theatres, car seat-belts, bicycles, narrow stairs, turnstiles, public changing rooms and toilet cubicles. Difficulties travelling on aeroplanes because of the size of the seats or seat-belts sometimes pose problems for people who are expected to travel by air for work (Longhurst 2005; Brandon and Pritchard 2011). Hetrick and Attig (2009) give the example of fat students who are required to sit in standard-size desks. They experience physical and emotional pain because of attempting to squeeze their larger bodies into too tight a space and the feelings of humiliation and shame this public mortification of the flesh inspires. Fat bodies which are too big to be comfortably inserted into standard-sized desks find themselves literally contained within rigid spatial boundaries that refuse to accommodate them comfortably:

> To sit in these desks – primarily in chairs attached to individual writing surfaces, or auditorium seating with hinged desks – our hips and stomachs must be pushed, shoved, and squeezed into unforgiving metal, wood, and plastic. The longer we sit in them, the more uncomfortable they become, biting into fleshy abundance and often resisting attempted release.
>
> *(Hetrick and Attig 2009: 197)*

From a Foucauldian perspective, such constraint of fat bodies is part of the disciplinary gaze and surveillance that attempts to normalize and control bodies that are considered excessive and out-of-control. When others are able to view the bodily movements of fat people in space, their attempts to fit into spaces too small for them, this gaze of others becomes part of the apparatus of power that both produces the figure of the fat body and attempts to regulate it (Longhurst 2005; Murray 2008; Hetrick and Attig 2009; Huff 2009). The doctor's surgery, for example, is a pivotal site in which surveillance, the disciplinary gaze and the moral censure of fat people regularly takes place. Fat people are incited to confess to the doctor the lifestyle choices that they have made, or their failure to follow medical guidelines concerning weight loss, as part of the pathologizing of fatness. It is impossible for fat people to avoid this line of questioning about their bodily habits because their fatness is so visible to the doctor. As Murray (2008, 2009a) has observed, when she has consulted a doctor her fatness has invariably been nominated by the doctor as the reason for her ailments.

Doctors repeatedly advised her to lose weight, because her 'obese' body was automatically positioned as problematic. She was expected to confess the pathology of her body mass, to demonstrate to the doctor that she was aware of the deviant nature of her body.

So too, going out into public spaces can be confronting for fat people, as they feel the assessing gazes of others upon their bodies, particularly in places where flesh is on display, such as beaches and swimming pools. Research with fat people has identified the shame they may feel about their bodies, and the social humiliation to which they are often exposed by others. For example, one man from the north of England spoke about his emotional distress at being laughed at by some young men while sitting in the sun in his shorts on holiday because of his fat body: 'they could see me and they were laughing and joking and carrying on and it was only as they got past that I realised that they were laughing at me, about how fat I was. And er, I mean it hurts' (quoted in Brandon and Pritchard 2011: 87). This feeling of self-consciousness about one's body is dynamic, subject to change depending on the social and cultural context in which individuals find themselves: 'In Asia I feel colossal and find myself continually clenching my body in an attempt to take up less space, but in the Pacific Islands, surrounded by larger-bodied people, I feel more relaxed' (Longhurst 2005: 253).

Fat people have not only observed others watching and assessing their own bodies, but have acknowledged that they themselves participate in making judgemental evaluations of other fat people and whether or not they should expose their flesh. As one woman commented: 'I know people go into, wear swimming costumes on the beach when they are my size, but [laughing] they shouldn't. Uh, you see, I'm, I'm fat and I can look at other people and say "oh, no, you shouldn't"' (quoted in Tischner and Malson 2008: 263). Fat people are not only the subjects of the surveilling and disciplinary gaze, therefore, but are also themselves implicated in this gaze by turning it upon other people as well as upon themselves.

Going supermarket shopping or eating in public are particularly emotionally fraught experiences for fat people because of the assumed link between food intake and fat embodiment. Fat people have commented on how strangers will inspect their shopping trolleys when shopping for food, as if to ascertain for themselves why that person is fat (Tischner and Malson 2008). When eating out, fat people may feel intensely self-conscious about the kind and amount of food they are eating in front of others. They may be subjected to comments from others (even strangers) questioning whether they should allow themselves to eat sweet treats, fried foods or large meals. If a fat person attempts to hide her eating from other people because of the shame she feels at being the object of their judgemental gaze, then she is viewed as indulging in food secretively as part of compulsive or addictive behaviour (Murray 2008: 59) in much the same way as the bulimic hides her food bingeing and purging from others.

Such assumptions render it difficult for a fat person to eat in any situation, public or private, without self-consciously feeling the assessing gaze upon him. Even if a fat person was viewed eating food that is accepted as healthy, or low-fat, that individual would still be subjected to assumptions concerning his fatness: that he was 'on a diet', for example, or trying to look as if he were eating 'properly' in public but might be indulging himself in private. Eating in public for fat people, therefore, can never be divorced from cultural expectations about the relationship between the fat body and indulgence and the need for self-discipline. As a result, fat women in particular rarely allow themselves to indulge in eating, as the notion of them as 'food addicts' suggests. Instead, they experience continual self-restraint and policing of their food intake in their attempts to conform to cultural expectations around body size and appropriate dietary consumption (Tischner and Malson 2008; Murray 2008, 2009a).

Fatness: a disability?

The notion of fatness as a disability has received some attention in critical approaches to obesity discourse. As I explained in Chapter 1, like contemporary fat activists, activists adopting the social model of disability argue that disability is experienced via the social and cultural meanings which surround it, as well as the materiality of the physical space in which people with disabilities must operate. Critical disability activists and scholars thus seek to counter negative and stigmatizing perspectives on disability and agitate for social change and improvement of facilities for people with disabilities.

Some commentators have compared the experience of having a fat body to that of having a physical disability, because the physical environment is structured so that both fat bodies and bodies with disabilities have difficulties moving around and being accommodated (Cooper 1997; Chan and Gillick 2009; Huff 2009; Aphramor 2009; Brandon and Pritchard 2011). Just as some disability activists assert that the spaces in which they are forced to move effectively contribute to their disability because their embodiment is not catered for, so too some fat activists point out that public space is not conducive to fat embodiment. The question of how much space fat bodies need on aeroplanes, for example, and whether they should be required to pay for an additional seat when flying, concerns debate about 'how much space a body can inhabit in an environment constructed by twenty-first century corporations' (Huff 2009: 184).

In making her argument that fatness should be regarded as a disability, Cooper (1997: 33) claims that, at least at the time in which she was writing, fat politics was seen as a 'little more than a joke' by people in the mainstream because the problems faced by fat people were viewed as trivial compared to those endured by people with disabilities. In response to this, she contends that labelling themselves as 'disabled' helps fat people to be taken more seriously and to emphasize the difficulties they face as ostracized and stigmatized members of society. There are many similarities between the mainstream sociocultural response to fat bodies and to those with disabilities. Both forms of embodiment are marginalized, discriminated against, viewed as differing from the norm, invisible, lacking and deficient, as a bodily state to be strenuously avoided. Both fat people and people with disabilities tend to be portrayed as objects of pity. The embodiment of both groups is viewed as requiring medical treatment. As noted above, like many people with disabilities, fat people find physical spaces difficult to negotiate and are 'disabled' by the lack of accommodation to their bodily differences. Indeed in several western countries, such as the United States, the United Kingdom, Canada and Sweden, fat people are given protection against discrimination under acts of legislation directed broadly at all kinds of disabilities or impairments which are viewed as limiting major life activities (Chan and Gillick 2009).

The major difference between the treatment of and attitudes towards fat people and people with disabilities is the notion that people with disabilities 'cannot help it' whereas fat people are to blame for their condition, something that they can change if they only 'tried hard enough' (Cooper 2007; Chan and Gillick 2009). Therefore malicious comments directed at fat people and drawing attention to their weight are often tolerated, whereas the same is generally not true of people with disabilities. Indeed people with disabilities who are not themselves fat may themselves have internalized negative views of fat people, including the notion that fatness is self-inflicted and not a result of ill fortune, like disability (Cooper 2007).

Fat people, for their part, may take exception to positioning themselves as disabled because of the stigmatizing meanings around this bodily difference and because they do not identify as disabled. One study involving interviews with seven American fat people (Chan and Gillick 2009) found that they were unwilling to adopt a disability identity based on their fatness. The participants were divided about the level of responsibility they attributed to fat embodiment. Most tended to see their fatness as hereditary, and therefore a condition beyond their individual control, or else caused by some other factor such as illness, psychological problems, psychiatric conditions or metabolic features. However they also spoke about attempting to lose weight by dieting or exercising. The interviewees therefore tended not to position their fatness as a disability because of the role played by choice in the condition. Even those people in the study who were willing to position themselves as disabled because of other conditions that they had, such as arthritis, diabetes or a psychiatric condition, were reluctant to identify fatness as a disability.

6

REFRAMING FAT

Fat activism and size acceptance politics

The previous chapter focused on the negative experiences many fat people endure as part of their everyday living of fat embodiment. This chapter, in contrast, discusses positive aspects and representations of fatness, particularly in the context of fat activism, which has attempted to disrupt and counter the hegemonic meanings surrounding fat embodiment.

Fat, out and proud

Many fat women, and to a lesser extent, men, and particularly those who identify with fat acceptance politics, have 'come out' as fat and have sought to represent fat bodies in positive ways. They claim that fatness need not be experienced as an unattractive or unhealthy state, and that by reclaiming the word 'fat' and taking steps to present themselves in positive and powerful ways, the dominant negative meanings around fat embodiment may be challenged and usurped. For fat activists and those advocating size acceptance, therefore, embodiment can be resignified and therefore reconstituted via discursive and political challenges to current discourses around fatness. They assert that while the 'fat body' in its fleshiness will not melt away through political and discursive resistant and subversive actions, changing the meanings around this flesh will change the experience of living in a fat body.

Fat activism began to emerge in the United States in the late 1960s as part of a turn towards politicizing structural inequality and mobilizing for civil rights in other marginalized social groups, such as women, gay men and lesbians and blacks. 'The Fat Liberation Manifesto' written by members of the Fat Underground contended that fat people should be treated with respect and have equal rights, and called for the ending of 'fat oppression' (Solovay and Rothblum 2009: 4). Since then, and particularly in response to the 'obesity epidemic' discourse emerging in the late 1990s, fat activism has gathered momentum, although with some notable exceptions it has largely been confined to the North American context (Johnston and Taylor 2008; Cooper 2009).

The American organization the National Association to Advance Fat Acceptance is the dominant fat acceptance group globally. It works to challenge structural discrimination against fat bodies by lobbying airlines and cinemas, for example, to make their seats wider and calling for legislation to counter fat discrimination in the workplace. Other activist groups include the Canadian-based Pretty, Porky, and Pissed Off, a grassroots organization formed by feminist and queer artists and activists in 1996, whose members engaged in public demonstrations and performances to highlight discrimination against fat people and to present fat bodies as sexually desirable and attractive (Johnston and Taylor 2008). In England The Chubsters has been formed, a group of self-proclaimed fat women who humorously represent themselves as members of a girl gang who are out to attack people for such behaviours as harassing fat people, insisting that fatness is unhealthy and boasting about their diets and gym memberships. A range of alternative media have provided alternative views on fat bodies, including independently produced magazines (or 'zines' as they are known) such as *FaT GiRl: A Zine for Fat Dykes and Women Who Want Them* and *Size Queen: For Queen Size Queers and Our Loyal Subjects* (Snider 2009). The latter type of fat activism represents a diversity of body types and sexual orientations and practices.

The internet has provided a major impetus to fat activist activities, allowing ready access to contesting views on fatness, from pornographic sites for people who have a sexual fetish for fat people, including heterosexual, gay and lesbian-oriented pornographic images, to a multitude of self-help sites, discussion groups and blogs recounting fat people's personal experiences. The internet allows fat activists to easily disseminate information about their cause and assists their mobilization for social action. Fat activist blogs are numerous, with names such as Big Fat Blog, Fat Chicks Rule, Fierce, Freethinking Fatties, Fatties United! and Feed Me! The typical format of such sites includes an 'About' section which presents the contributors, describes their experiences as a fat person and details their fat acceptance political position. Many such blogs include updates of debates in the expert literature on the health effects of obesity or critiques of public health campaigns about obesity or news media reporting.

Erotic and pornographic images have also been produced which seek to represent fat men and women as actively sexual and attractive, as in the zines described above and in more mainstream magazines and websites. There is a specialist type of pornography that features very fat women which shows these women eating in the nude or semi-clad rather than engaging in sexual activity. The predominant erotic focus is on their fleshy stomachs and food entering a fat woman's mouth. Gay pornographic websites and magazines also feature fat men – so-called 'chubby porn'. There are also sites for heterosexuals featuring 'Big Handsome Men' and 'Bears' (who tend to be both fat and hirsute), some of whom focus on the pleasure of feeding men ('Gainers' or 'Belly Builders') to promote weight gain as part of erotic practice (Kulick 2005; Monaghan 2005b). In addition several performance-oriented groups, particularly in the United States, have been formed which seek to represent fat women in sensual and erotic ways, including fat burlesque performers or strippers and fat belly dancers, with names such as Big Burlesque, the Glamazon Girls and the Corpulent Cuties.

Naturally fat?

One dominant argument in the fat activist literature concerns the issue of personal responsibility for fatness. Many fat activist writers contend that fat embodiment is not a 'lifestyle choice', as is generally presented by the anti-obesity perspective, but rather a product of a combination of genetic and other physiological factors which work together to ensure that their bodies are very efficient at storing fat tissue. Fatness is therefore represented as an inherent physical attribute, like gender, skin colour, race or sexual orientation. These writers assert that fat people are not fat because they eat more than others or exercise less, or in any other way behave in a self-indulgent, greedy or lazy manner (Burgard *et al.* 2009; Wann 2009). Thus, for example, Wann contends that 'Plenty of people think that I choose to be fat' and goes on to seek to prove that her fat embodiment is not her choice at all. She asserts that the current dominant belief that body weight is a product of personal choice about lifestyle is 'a big, fat lie'. Wann argues that she does not over-eat and regularly engages in exercise, and yet is still fat because 'nature is stronger than nurture' (2005: 61).

It is asserted by these writers that fatness is merely one end of a normal spectrum of body size. Wann (2009) goes on to argue that just as the height range of individuals follows a bell curve, ranging from very short to extremely tall, so too there is a diversity of body weight, from very thin to fat. She again uses

the term 'natural' in describing this diversity of height and
weight to imply that biological variance is inherently a feature
of bodily diversity. While access to resources such as food and
medicine may have an influence on body size, '[t]here have
always been and will always be people of different heights. There
have also always been and there will also always be people of
different weights' (Wann 2009: x).

Such approaches to fat, therefore, adopt a scientific essential-
ism similar to that offered by the orthodox medical perspective.
While writers using this approach challenge the assertions
about fat put forward by mainstream obesity science, they draw
selectively upon alternative medical theories on obesity to support their assertions. Their bodies are 'naturally fat' because of a
biological propensity to gain weight, and therefore should not be
negatively judged for their size. There are strong parallels in such
arguments with those put forward by some gay activists, who
have long contended that same-sex attraction (or bisexuality, or
transgender identity) is not a choice, but rather a biological
imperative. One is born gay or lesbian, one is not made gay
or lesbian, goes the common and well-rehearsed argument.
Divergence from the normative body size, therefore, should be
accepted not only based on the liberal championing of diversity
but also because of the realization that fatness (like sexual orientation) is genetically inherent.

Similarly, the Health at Every Size (HAES) movement positions itself in direct opposition to the dominant discourses of
obesity science by directing attention away from fatness and
the aim of losing weight to a focus on the importance of
health regardless of body size. At its title suggests, the HAES
movement encourages valuing diversity of body size and weight
and celebrating every type of body without making value
judgements about which kind of body is 'healthy' or not. It
involves a focus on achieving good health, and preventing ill-
health and disease, but avoiding too great a restrictive emphasis
on controlling food intake. It emphasizes the 'pleasure' of eating

and the 'joy' of moving one's body, so as to counter the dominant messages of health promotional and commodity culture's portrayals of health in relation to body weight. The goal, therefore, is to focus on achieving good health, without paying attention to body weight (Burgard 2009; Aphramor and Gringas 2011).

The BMI is wholeheartedly rejected by the HAES movement for a notion of the body as having an individual 'natural' weight at which it is healthiest. Some proponents of this approach argue that individuals have a weight range to which their bodies are physiologically predisposed (and this set point will vary from person to person), above or below which they will experience ill health. The goal is to keep within the set-weight range by engaging in healthy eating and exercise habits.

Here again, the body in this discourse is portrayed as a natural phenomenon. Individuals will be able to tell instinctively from how they feel whether or not they are eating well enough or moving their bodies enough. The ideal of 'nurturing the body' rather than punishing it or controlling it in the attempt to lose weight is presented. People are encouraged to listen to their body's cues to determine whether or not to eat a particular food, or whether they are hungry or full. Health is defined as 'the process of daily life rather than the outcome of weight' (Burgard 2009: 44). Thus, the HAES approach contends that at any given weight, some people are healthy and some are not, depending on a wide range of variables, both physiological and environmental.

Ethics and feminist fat politics

Some academic writers have deemed it vital to their personal, political and academic projects to 'come out' in their academic writing as fat people, or at the very least, as accepting of fat embodiment. The association between feminist critiques of fatness and fat acceptance politics is so strong that it is some-times very difficult for feminist writers to acknowledge that they may wish to lose weight themselves. In an article published in the feminist philosophy journal *Hypatia*, for example, Ann Cahill wrote of her struggles with her feminist identity and her decision to take action to lose weight:

> I have become one of those people: Someone Who Has Lost Weight. Even more, I'm rapidly becoming another kind of person: Someone Who Has Lost Weight and Kept It Off. There are some for whom this kind of identity would be nothing more than welcome, but for me, a feminist and a philosopher, it can feel like an ill-fitting coat.
>
> *(Cahill 2010: 485–86)*

Cahill (2010: 486) went on to note that 'From the beginning, the question of purpose was crucial. What did I, as a feminist woman, have to gain from changing my relationship to food?' She justified her decision to cut down on her food intake and engage in a regular exercise programme in the attempt to lose weight as based on the desire to feel physically strong rather than attempting to conform to stereotypical notions of female attractiveness or even for health reasons. Her goal in losing weight was 'maximizing my ability to *move*, quickly, effectively, strongly ... I wanted to bring strength and vigor to whatever struggle I chose. I wanted to get to my fighting weight' (2010: 486, original emphasis).

This focus on strength rather than slimness – indeed, in direct contrast to what Cahill (2010: 486) described as the 'frailty' of 'skinniness' – allowed her to engage in significant weight reduc-tion, at the same time as she built physical fitness and muscular strength from her running and weight training exercise pro-gramme, and to continue to feel as if she had not contravened her feminist principles. She argued that her scholarly training as a feminist philosopher allowed her to engage in these bodily practices in a state that was highly aware of the pitfalls of descending into hatred of her body or fear of food, and to position these practices as about strength and quality of life rather than about beauty or demonstrating self-control over the unruly body. Cahill asserts that she never identified as 'fat' and never felt repulsed by her body. Instead she saw her previously 'larger' body simply as 'different' from the one she achieved through her weight-loss programme.

Another ethical conundrum for feminists who are committed to the principles and ideas of size acceptance and fat activism is bariatric surgery, a practice of which many fat activists have been extremely critical. They have typically represented such surgical interventions as a grotesque 'mutilation' of the body, a radical procedure aimed at 'curing' a bodily state (fatness) which they do not accept as posing a risk to their health. Indeed, choosing to undergo this surgery would be tantamount to accepting the orthodox biomedical assumptions that 'obesity' is a disease and poses an extreme health risk, and repudiating the idea that bodies of any size should be accepted without judgement.

Samantha Murray is an Australian feminist cultural studies writer who has based her academic writing around fat acceptance and theorizing the cultural meanings of fatness for women (see, for example, Murray 2005, 2008, 2009a, 2009b). She has published several critiques of the ways in which fat women's bodies are subjected to moralistic and judgemental assumptions, and written insightfully about the experiences of being a fat woman. She has also written critically of the ways in which her own fat body and those of other fat people are inevitably viewed by doctors as pathological and at risk of disease because of their fatness (see Chapter 5). Yet, after some years of contributing to the literature and politics of size acceptance and fat studies, Murray chose the extremely radical action of undergoing bariatric surgery herself.

Murray (2009b) writes that while she remained politically committed to the fat liberation movement and to the ideals of size diversity, she still struggled in her everyday embodied life with being fat. When Murray found that she was experiencing continuing ill health, and was diagnosed with severe insulin resistance, polycystic ovarian syndrome and hormone imbalances, she was advised by her doctor to conform to a medical and dietary regime. When, after a year, her condition had not improved, her doctor recommended that she have a gastric band implanted in her stomach. She notes that this suggestion made her 'furious', as it contravened so many of her own political ideals, and she felt that these would be compromised by undergoing the surgery. Further, as noted above, Murray had previously written pieces highly critical of medicine's tendency to suggest that fatness leads to ill health. Yet she was now forced to concede that her own fatness was causing serious health problems and to agree to undergo a surgical procedure of which she had been highly critical.

I thought about similar issues when writing this book. Not because I am fat or have ever sought to lose weight, but because I have always been thin and have never struggled with body weight issues. I wondered as I researched and wrote this book whether I would be open to criticism on the part of fat activists for my inability to join the sisterhood of abundant flesh and write from lived experience, as many of them do. Nonetheless, I would claim that to argue that only self-professed fat people should be able to write critically about fatness is misguided. Indeed it could be argued that for fat people to exclude people who do not conform to or identify with this form of embodiment is to engage in the kind of exclusion based on body type which they themselves critique. Indeed, while some fat activists are rather dismissive of non-fat people writing about fat issues (see, for example, Cooper 2010), as I noted in Chapter 1 others have made the point that all individuals, regardless of body size or weight, are affected in some way by the power of obesity discourse.

Further, it is not only fat people who are explicitly targeted and affected by obesity discourses. As discussed in Chapter 3, mothers of young children have also found themselves subjected to moralizing and guilt-inducing imperatives in obesity policy, health promotion campaigns and mass media representations of the 'childhood obesity problem'. Cooper (2010) has argued that the perspectives of fat people themselves have often been absent in academic research on fatness/obesity. So too, I would argue, the voices of mothers with young children have not often received attention, except when researchers want to determine how well they are conforming to advice on controlling their children's weight. Whether these women are themselves fat or not, they have been charged with the responsibility of dealing with or preventing fat in their children's bodies, a position which is highly morally and emotionally charged. This is something of which I do have direct experience, as a mother of two school-aged girls who juggles her own feminist and ethical principles with attempting to promote her daughters' health and emotional wellbeing.

There are many difficult ethical questions to negotiate when dealing with children and weight control as a mother. How do mothers ensure that their children are healthy without instilling a hatred and fear of fat or of their own body if they do not conform to the ideal of slim embodiment? How do they deal with resistance on the part of their children when they are reluctant to eat healthy foods or exercise according to official guidelines? How do mothers deal with children's comments that they feel that they are 'too fat'? Should mothers of fat children encourage these children to engage in the 'fat pride' espoused by fat activism and give up attempts to encourage them to lose weight, and by doing so directly counter the neoliberal expectations of 'good motherhood'? These are all difficult issues at the heart of family life with young or adolescent children in the context of the intensification of public discourse on the 'childhood obesity crisis' and the responsibility bestowed upon mothers for promoting the optimal health and development of their children in all aspects of their lives.

Critiques of fat activism

While fat activism and mainstream feminist approaches to fatness are widely accepted within critical weight studies and fat studies, there are a number of points of debate and criticism of these perspectives which need to be acknowledged. As I have noted, the predominant proponents of fat activism or size acceptance are feminist women who themselves identify as fat. This itself tends to exclude consideration of other people's experiences in relation to obesity discourse. I made the point above that it is not only fat women who are discriminated against or incited to feel guilt and shame by hegemonic obesity discourse. Just as mothers' experiences have been little examined, the experiences of fat children have rarely been addressed.

One could also question where the fat male body fits within this feminist and activist literature on fatness. Feminist and activist writings almost exclusively focus on the implications for fat female bodies of obesity discourse. Far less scholarship and research has been published on the implications for fat male bodies. Far fewer forums exist for fat men to challenge the negative meanings of male fatness, to attempt to represent it positively or to receive support as members of a stigmatized outgroup. So too, the fat activist literature has been thus far been dominated by an American-centric focus, with little discussion of whether arguments from this geographical location may be relevant to other western countries, and particularly to non-western countries (Cooper 2009).

Another interesting question for fat activism and fat identity is whether attempts to reclaim the term 'fat' and use it as a means of joining a particular oppressed minority group is to posit an essentialist position on fatness. This position is challenged by those writing from a queer studies perspective, who see identities not as fixed (as in the essentialist 'biologically fat body' posited by many fat activists) but as constantly shifting, requiring performative and constitutive acts to bring identity into being (Butler 1990; Sedgwick 1990; LeBesco 2001). Indeed the idea that everyone at some stage in their lives 'feels fat' in a 'fat-phobic society' is a nod to the notion that fat identities are constantly mutable, both within the same person and across the diversity of human embodiment and experience.

The fat activist perspective has been subjected to critique on the part of other feminists, including those who identify as fat and activists. Murray (2005, 2008), for example, is concerned that fat activism tends to focus on the individual by emphasizing the importance of fat people changing the way in which they think about themselves. Such individualistic approaches, she asserts, contribute to a splitting of mind and body, whereby fat people are encouraged to 'love themselves' despite their fat embodiment: to use the power of their minds to change the way they feel about themselves. She uses Merleau-Ponty's concept of 'being-in-the-world' to contend that such a split between mind and body is not ontologically possible, given that all human experience is always inevitably embodied. Murray points out that other people's responses and reactions to fat people are equally as important, and indeed constitutive, of how fat people think about their bodies/selves. As much as an individual fat person may work hard to think of his or her body in positive ways, others' responses will constantly challenge these ways of thinking if they remain negative.

Murray (2005, 2008) also argues that the size acceptance movement tends to assume a self that is amenable to rational action and change based on knowledge, and therefore privileges the mind, assuming its dominance over and distinction from, the fleshly body. This perspective on selfhood assumes a unitary 'fat self' which fat people are encouraged to militantly celebrate when they 'come out as fat'. Such a 'proud fat self' is not able to concede that she or he may sometimes dislike being fat.

Ambivalence about fat pride is not encouraged or accepted in fat activist discourse, for it is seen as giving in to the prevailing negative discourses around fat embodiment. In contrast, Murray wants to emphasize the potential for ambiguity and ambivalence in fat politics: to acknowledge that fat people, however hard they try, may not quite manage to 'think themselves' positive about their fat embodiment and may have to struggle with feelings of ambivalence about their fatness or even openly to confront their own self-hatred and disgust about their body or other fat bodies. Fat people, she contends have 'complicated and tacit investments' in the discourses and practices which construct them as fat subjects even as they seek to resist or counter these discourses and practices (Murray 2008: 90).

As this suggests, fat people cannot ever extricate themselves from the network of meaning, discourse, practice, material objects and other bodies in which they live and experience their bodies. They are assemblages of all these phenomena which configure their bodies and selves. Fat people cannot force other people to see fat embodiment as positive, even if they themselves insist upon this way of seeing. Size acceptance groups, however, often advocate that fat people should dissociate their 'real selves' from the fat flesh encasing them, so that they can feel valued for these selves. They are encouraged to look beyond their bodies to value the qualities within. At the same time, however, fat pride also encourages fat people to give positive meanings to their fat embodiment, to see fat as attractive, normal and healthy rather than ugly and pathological (Murray 2008). Murray (2008) notes that there is a central contradiction here between on the one hand wanting to value a self apart from, and dwelling 'inside', the body and on the other wanting to give value to the body itself which bespeaks an ambivalence about fatness. She calls instead for a recognition and acceptance of ambiguity of subjectivity, a crucial move which acknowledges the dynamic, unfinished and heterogeneous dimensions of selfhood and embodiment.

Probyn (2008) has also criticized fat activism's focus on positive representations of the fat body in popular culture to the exclusion of other issues. She notes that insisting on a 'semiotic reversal' (2008: 402), in which meanings around fatness are countered and negated for other meanings, and 'fat becomes objectified as a mode of resistance' (2008: 403), does not challenge the political and social structuring underpinnings of obesity discourse and fat embodiment. Like other writers who have observed that fat activism and critical weight studies too often limit their focus to identifying and critiquing discourse and representation (Guthman and DuPuis 2006), she calls for a more material analysis, in which the systems of agribusiness producing and marketing poor quality foods and the damage to people's health caused by the type of food they eat are acknowledged and singled out for critique.

These critics argue that fat activists may have to accept that to some extent fat embodiment may not be a cause for celebration: that it may sometimes have negative physical effects that need to be acknowledged (as Murray was forced to do by undergoing bariatric surgery). So too, the ramifications for people's health, whether or not they are fat, in relation to the economies of food production, distribution and marketing need to be highlighted. They assert that it is one thing to identify and challenge the discriminatory attitudes to which fat people are exposed, but it is quite another to deny that there are any kinds of material inconvenience or suffering associated with the lived experience of being fat or in eating poor quality foods which are detrimental to good health. Indeed I would contend that the rampant individualism and rejection of anti-obesity strictures evident in some fat activist discourses, which claim that people should be able to eat what they like and be able to grow to whatever body size they wish, is similar in many ways to the 'free choice' discourse offered by libertarian sceptics (Chapter 2), who are anxious to campaign against government measures against the production, marketing and consumption of poor quality foods by invoking the 'nanny state' argument.

In yet another perspective on this debate, Kirkland (2011) posits a criticism of what she calls the 'environmental' account of obesity (and others entitle the 'obesogenic' model), by arguing that feminists like Probyn who draw attention to the structural causes of obesity tend to impose their white, middle-class values on the socioeconomically disadvantaged. Kirkland contends that while they are well-meaning, such attempts often veer very close to being intrusive, moralizing, patronizing and punitive, for they still expect members of underprivileged groups to make 'responsible choices' once supposed 'barriers to change' are removed. She asserts that such critiques fail to acknowledge the debate in the academic literature concerning the validity of obesity science (discussed in Chapter 2) and tend to simply accept the pronouncements and assumptions of orthodox medical and public health approaches to obesity.

The debate here, which is still very much in its infancy, is similar in some ways to that which has been operating among critical disability activists and scholars. As discussed in Chapter 5, some fat studies writers have compared the experiences of fat people with those of people with disabilities, and have employed the social model of disability as a means of explaining the lived experiences of fat embodiment. It is very difficult to counter the social model of fatness or disability: to argue, instead, that perhaps it needs to be acknowledged that the embodied experience of fatness may sometimes be onerous because of the sheer weight and size of the body. Yet as Shakespeare (2011) has remarked in relation to disability, quite apart from dealing with the discrimination to which people with disabilities may be subjected, on the level of the everyday experience of life sometimes it is frankly better not to have disabilities than to have to deal with the inconveniences, discomfort and sometimes the excruciating and chronic pain that disabilities may bring with them. This kind of statement is extremely controversial within critical disability studies, as is the equivalent statement one could make about fatness, particularly for feminists writing in the context of a liberal humanist critique within which it is constantly contended that acceptance of any type of bodily manifestation should be supported and encouraged. Yet these dissenting viewpoints need to be aired and debated openly. It will be interesting to observe how critical weight studies and fat studies deal with these critiques and debates as they mature and develop.

CONCLUDING COMMENTS

I end this book with some comments about how individuals have resisted the dominant imperatives issuing forth from obesity discourse, the question of whether the power of this discourse is beginning to dissipate, and the identification of major overarching themes emerging from the discussions in the book concerning the body, the self and medical power in contemporary western societies.

Resisting obesity discourse

One feature of Foucauldian writings on biopower and governmentality which has been subject to some criticism is the tendency of such perspectives to position individuals as constrained and manipulated by the imperatives championed by dominant institutions such as medicine, public health and the mass media. Yet, in the context of weight control, it is clear (if only from the large number of people designated as 'overweight' or 'obese' in western countries) that these imperatives are often not conformed to. Much to the chagrin of those employed in health promotional or medical efforts directed at weight control, many people apparently resist their suggestions to change their behaviours, despite the avalanche of warnings in both expert and popular forums about the risks associated with overweight and obesity. While people readily reproduce the dominant discourses espousing controlled and healthy eating and regular physical exercise in the interests of weight control and good health, they often also report failing to take up this advice. These constitute instances of what Walkerdine (2009: 205) describes as the 'unspoken other to the subject of biopower' – the resistant subject, or 'bodies who refuse to regulate themselves'.

What impels this resistance? It cannot be claimed that it is due to simple lack of knowledge, as is often assumed in public health research and health policy. The publicity around the 'obesity epidemic' and associated health promotional campaigns has been so pervasive that few people have missed the messages urging them to reduce their weight. Many people are making alternative choices, or perhaps they actively disagree with these expert discourses. They may be committed to alternative imperatives that counter or oppose those issuing from medical and public health advice, or have other interests or values which do not conform to the prevailing bourgeois ideal of the self-regulated subject seeking maximum health and longevity. They may resent being lectured to by state agencies or medical professionals about how they should conduct their everyday lives and having their freedom to do what they like curtailed.

Some people may simply prefer to be fat than thin. Because fat bodies are large bodies, they may impart a sense of solidity and substantialness to the fat person. Some fat men have recounted a feeling of power from having a very large body that takes up space, makes them noticed: this is evident in black rap culture, for example. In a cultural context in which small, slight men's bodies are considered effeminate or girlish, lacking traditional masculine power, at least the fat male body is solid and big.

Some fat women have also commented on the ways in which their fatness makes them feel noticed and gives them a sense of power in the workplace setting equivalent to a masculine sense of bodily empowerment and authority (Bell and McNaughton 2007; Tischner and Malson 2008, 2011). As the previous chapter showed, fat activists, for their part, have been extremely vocal and vehement in challenging dominant meanings around fatness and any suggestion that they should attempt to lose weight. So too, the concept of the 'fat bastard', as it is used by British working-class men, may constitute a form of resistance to the confining imperatives of obesity discourse when used in ways that demonstrate pride in this form of embodiment rather than shame, and as part of a membership of a similarly embodied group. The notions that 'everybody is different', that the BMI is just a number and people should judge for themselves how heavy they should be based on how they feel or what body type they have (Monaghan 2007; Evans and Colls 2009; Ristovski-Slijepcevic *et al.* 2010) are also ways in which people express their resistance to the normalizing imperatives of health education and mass media reporting of the relationship between body weight and health.

Emotional response is also an important dimension of how people respond to the regulative practices of biopower. Emotion may impel people's efforts to conform to dominant obesity discourses: their fear of looking unattractive, facing stigmatization, ridicule or disgust from others or developing a serious illness or dying young, or conversely, pleasure, pride and a feeling of accomplishment in losing weight and achieving an overtly disciplined, slim body. Health promotion campaigns routinely attempt to invoke these kinds of emotional response in their audiences to persuade them to take up weight control strategies. But emotion is also integral to resistance to biopedagogies. In the context of schools, for example, the boredom engendered by yet another attempt to teach the same old facts about the importance of exercise and healthy eating or resentment about being measured in public or having one's lunch box assessed for its healthiness (Evans *et al.* 2008; Evans and Colls 2009; Leahy 2009).

In the face of their positioning as responsible for monitoring and normalizing their own weight and that of their children, some mothers have chosen to resist these dominant meanings by positioning their ample body size as 'motherly' and 'cuddly', by contending that caring for their children is more important than worrying about their own body weight, and that preparing nourishing and satisfying meals for their families is more important than counting the calories in these meals (Warin *et al.* 2008; Fullagar 2009). As this suggests, many mothers view food provisioning and preparation for their children as an integral part of their loving relationship with them. While nutrition and weight issues are considered important, so also are the values of family togetherness and enjoyment, the emotional dimensions of love, nurturing and shared pleasure (Lupton 1996). These affective dimensions of mothers' caring work and family relationships tend to be ignored or else repudiated for their irrationality in official discourses on maternal responsibility for children's body weight and nutrition.

The affective relationship that people have with the food and drink they choose to consume is also vital in understanding why they may refuse to take up expert advice on weight control. Eating for many people is an extremely pleasurable dimension of their lives and an important way in which they allow themselves some self-indulgence. In interviews about food and health imperatives people often express their disdain for the asceticism required of them by weight control edicts. Food can be a form of release from the strictures and stresses of everyday life, a comfort and release from boredom or tension. The notions of 'guilty pleasure' or 'reward' are often employed in people's accounts of why they allow themselves food that is designated as 'unhealthy' or 'fattening' (Lupton 1996; Madden and Chamberlain 2010). The concept of 'negotiated pleasures' underpins many people's rationales for why they continue to eat such food, as it employs the idea that as long as one is eating other healthy foods the occasional treat is allowable (Jallinoja *et al.* 2010). Fat people have remarked upon enjoying the freedom to eat what they liked when not trapped within the surveilling and disapproving gaze of others, positioning unrestrained eating as a form of freedom and rebellion (Tischner and Malson 2011).

The continuing struggle between the ethics of rationality and self-control and the valorizing of the expression of and engagement with one's emotions and the indulging of one's bodily desires and impulses is evident in these ways of thinking about food. While the successful control of one's body in pursuit of good health and physical attractiveness has its own pleasures, so too does 'letting go' of rigid control, allowing hedonistic self-indulgence. The grotesque body, although always transgressive, is not always stigmatized. In certain moments, spaces and temporalities (for example, at home after a hard day's work, on special occasions such as Christmas, at the pub or a party on a Friday or Saturday night) many people allow themselves some degree of hedonistic transgression from the usual strictures they may impose upon themselves. This might include deliberate risk-taking which contravenes official medical or public health advice, such as smoking, binge-drinking and eating 'unhealthy' foods (Lupton 1995, 1996, 1999).

Here again the concept of bodily assemblages may be employed as a way of recognizing the complexity of the flows of affect, power relations, engagement with material objects, sensual experience and interpersonal relations which configure and reconfigure bodies. Whatever their size, people's concepts of their bodies are changeable, their idea of themselves as fat or otherwise is dynamic and highly contextual. While they may be receptive to the dominant biopedagogical messages about weight control on some occasions, on others these meanings are directly challenged or simply forgotten.

Expert obesity discourses, therefore, cannot easily or permanently territorialize bodies.

The end of the 'obesity epidemic'?

Sociologist Michael Gard claims in his most recent book, contentiously entitled *The End of the Obesity Epidemic* (2011), that by 2010 the concept of the 'obesity epidemic' had begun to lose resonance in medical and media forums. He argues that the global health crisis predicted by orthodox medical and public health authorities had not eventuated by 2010, and that by the late 2000s, news media interest began to wane. Gard speculates that perhaps the emergence of the global financial crisis in the late 2000s was a reason for the focus on fat to begin to dissipate. So too, the growing number of publications expressing the counter-claims of obesity sceptics may have had an impact by challenging and subverting the orthodox line on the obesity epidemic. The arguments of sceptics were largely ignored by the medical and public health establishment for some time. Nonetheless, by 2005 Gard argues that there began to be evidence of recognition that there existed dissenting views in this literature.

My own exploration of articles published in prestigious international medical journals from 2008 to 2011 certainly reveals evidence that some medical and public health researchers are aware of controversial and dissenting views, and reference critics such as Campos in their work. However, their response is largely to continue to argue against these and call for people to lose weight in the interests of their health. Statements such as 'we dispute claims that the current problem of obesity is being exaggerated' (Huang *et al.* 2009: 45) continue to be made constantly by those subscribing to the anti-obesity perspective. To further investigate the level of medical interest in obesity I undertook an analysis of articles mentioning obesity in the *British Medical Journal* from 1995 to 2011. I found that rather than

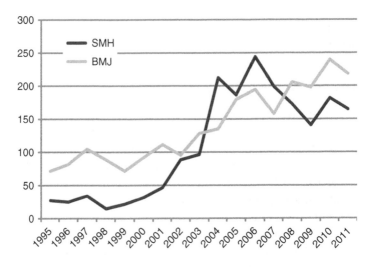

FIGURE 1 Obesity articles published in the *British Medical Journal* (BMJ) and *The Sydney Morning Herald* (SMH), 1995 to 2011.

interest in obesity on the part of medical researchers diminishing, as suggested by Gard, in terms of numbers of articles published there was evidence of a steadily growing interest, to the point that the greatest number of articles on obesity for any one year over that period was published in 2010 (see Figure 1).

It is perhaps inevitable that the news media would eventually lose interest in a specific health issue such as obesity, as it is difficult for journalists to sustain focus on an issue over a long period of time if there are no new angles on the story. It was certainly a feature of news reporting on HIV/AIDS that an initial extremely strong interest in the disease over several years in the 1980s dwindled to very little in the 1990s (Lupton 1994). HIV/AIDS is now a condition that receives very little news coverage, despite the fact that it continues to affect millions of people world-wide, particularly in some countries in Africa and Asia. While the focus on obesity in the news media may have peaked in the mid to late 2000s, news media reports continue to refer to the 'obesity epidemic' and repeat alarming speculations about the health risks of obesity and the growing numbers of obese people.

My own analysis of articles mentioning obesity published in the Australian broadsheet *The Sydney Morning Herald* from 1995 to 2011 found that while the numbers of articles peaked in 2006 and have decreased gradually since that time, there was still quite strong interest shown in the years following (Figure 1). More importantly, the content of the reports has remained the same, continually repeating concerns about the 'obesity epidemic' and the importance of people losing weight to avoid health problems, with little acknowledgement that the claims of obesity science may be contentious (see also Holland *et al.* 2011).

Governments in western countries have also continued to invest large sums to fund health promotion campaigns seeking to counter obesity, suggesting that politicians and policy makers have not responded to sceptical views on obesity and continue to position it as a major health problem in need of major intervention. For example, the American 'Let's Move' campaign, directed at controlling childhood obesity, was launched by First Lady Michelle Obama in early 2010, while on the same day President Obama created a Taskforce on Childhood Obesity. The Australian 'Swap It, Don't Stop It' anti-obesity campaign commenced in early 2011. For these reasons, I think that to pronounce that the power of the 'obesity epidemic' discourse has significantly lessened is somewhat premature.

Wider implications of obesity discourse

Finally, I end this book with some comments about the wider implications of the arguments here presented. While this book has focused on obesity discourse and fat embodiment, it may be asserted that these can be viewed as exemplars – albeit currently very potent ones – of the ways in which contemporary western societies think about and deal with illness, disease, health-related risks and the body. Obesity discourse is a powerful way of representing and configuring bodies that has achieved prominence at this point in history, eclipsing, for example, the panic engendered by HIV/AIDS in the 1980s or the SARS pandemic in the early 2000s.

Analysis of the way in which obesity discourse has achieved this power has revealed certain themes about how we currently conceptualize and attempt to control bodies. These include the following:

- The power of scientific medicine to construct definitions around bodies which distinguish between 'the normal' and 'the pathological'.
- The importance placed upon taking responsibility for one's health and making 'wise choices' as an entrepreneurial citizen in neoliberal societies.
- The state's use of biopedagogical strategies to inform citizens about their responsibilities in disciplining their consumption in the context of a political environment in which enthusiastic consumption is also encouraged.
- The continuing dialectic between the ascetic imperatives of disciplining consumption to ensure a healthy body and the pleasures of consumption as part of the hedonistic enjoyment of life.
- The growing use of measurement technologies to produce a virtual body assemblage comprised of data on 'risk factors'.
- The conflation of the concept of health with those of physical attractiveness, slim embodiment and personal accomplishment.
- The moral meanings which link lack of self-discipline with illness and disease.
- The disgust and abjection inspired by the ill, diseased or otherwise non-normative body.

- The construction of concepts of Self and Other in relation to the body and its perceived control of body boundaries and fluidities.
- The privileging of the tightly controlled, hard, impermeable body as the ideal to which other bodies are encouraged to aspire.

These features of how we think and feel about bodies go well beyond debates concerning the 'obesity epidemic'. They raise fundamental questions about the nature of embodiment and subjectivity in contemporary western societies and the role played by medicine and public health in constructing moral categories, regulating and giving meaning to bodies and disciplining or punishing Otherness.

GLOSSARY OF KEY TERMS

Abjection the phenomenon of being deemed 'abject' or provoking feelings of uneasiness, disgust, fear and revulsion due to liminal status, blurring the boundaries between Self and Other.

Assemblage the dynamic body/self produced by the interaction of an individual's body with other bodies, non-human living organisms, material objects, discourse, practices, space and place.

Bariatric surgery surgical techniques designed to achieve major weight loss, such as gastric banding or other means of reducing stomach size and capacity.

Bio-citizen a mode of citizenship produced through processes of bodily monitoring, surveillance and regulation and expectations about individual responsibility for maintaining good health.

Biopedagogies educational practices that are directed at instructing people how to conduct, regulate and discipline their bodies.

Biopolitics the disciplining and monitoring of individuals by the state via practices, regulations and discourses directed at the body, both at the individual and the population level.

Biopower the operation of power relations through and with the body.

Body Mass Index (BMI) a mathematical calculation of body weight produced by dividing an individual's weight by the square of that person's height. The resultant BMI is then compared against a chart which gives guidelines for the cut-off points designating individuals as 'underweight', 'normal weight', 'overweight' or 'obese'.

Culture-bound syndrome a disease or condition that is specific to a belief system operating in a particular cultural or geographical context.

Discourse a defined and coherent way of representing and discussing people, events or things, as expressed in a range of forums, from everyday talk to the popular media and the internet to expert talk and texts.

Globesity the spread of obesity and overweight around the world.

Governmentality a system of government by which the state encourages citizens to take responsibility for their own health and wellbeing voluntarily rather than being coerced.

Medicalization the process by which phenomena are defined as illnesses, diseases or conditions requiring medical intervention.

Neoliberalism a political approach evident in contemporary western societies which is characterized by an emphasis on citizens' opportunities to make free choices, albeit guided in certain ways by the state, and which promotes the concept of citizens voluntarily seeking to take responsibility for their own health and welfare.

Obesity the medical term for an individual's body mass that exceeds a BMI of 29.

Obesity discourse the conglomeration of official or expert ways of talking about and representing fat bodies from a medicalized perspective.

Obesogenic environment the combination of social structural factors believed to encourage the over-consumption of food and a sedentary lifestyle, thus leading to overweight or obesity.

Overweight the medical term for a BMI between 25 and 29.

Poststructuralism a theoretical perspective drawn principally from the writings of French philosophers, including Foucault, Deleuze and Guattari, and Kristeva, which is interested in the constitution of bodies and selves via language and discourse and which emphasizes the contingent, hybrid and performative nature of bodies and selves.

Territorialization the dynamic process by which interactions of humans and non-humans take place within, through and between spaces and places.

WEBLIOGRAPHY

The Adipositivity Project (http://adipositivity.com): displays visual images of fat bodies presented in positive ways which seek to widen definitions of physical beauty.

Big Fat Blog (http://www.bigfatblog.com): one of the best-known sites devoted to fat acceptance politics.

The Chubsters (http://www.chubstergang.com): an English-based group of female fat activists.

Fat Culture (http://pinterest.com/dalupton/fat-culture): a collection of images depicting the social and cultural dimensions of fat embodiment.

Fat Dialogue (http://www.fatdialogue.com): an interactive fat studies hub moderated by Australian fat activist and scholar Samantha Murray.

Health at Every Size (http://haescommunity.org): a website devoted to the movement which emphasizes the importance of promoting health regardless of body weight or size.

International Size Acceptance Association (www.size-acceptance.org)

National Association to Advance Fat Acceptance (www.naafa.org)

Obesity Time Bomb (http://www.obesitytimebomb.blogspot.com): British fat activist and scholar Charlotte Cooper's blog.

BIBLIOGRAPHY

Anonymous (2010) '21 celebrities that got fat'. Online. Available: http://damncoolpictures.com/2010/06/21-celebrities-that-got-fat.html (accessed 9 January 2012).
—— (2012) 'The Biggest Loser'. Online. Available: http://en.wikipedia.org/wiki/The_Biggest_Loser (accessed 2 January 2012).
Aphramor, L. (2005) 'Is a weight-centred health framework saluto-genic? Some thoughts on unhinging certain dietary ideologies', *Social Theory & Health*, 3(4): 315–40.
—— (2009) 'Disability and the anti-obesity offensive', *Disability & Society*, 24(7): 897–909.
Aphramor, L. and Gringas, J. (2008) 'Sustaining imbalance – evidence of neglect in the pursuit of traditional nutritional health', in S. Riley, M. Burns, H. Frith, S. Wiggins and P. Markula (eds) *Critical Bodies: Representations, Identities and Practices of Weight and Body Management*, Houndmills: Palgrave Macmillan, 155–74.
—— (2011) 'Helping people change: promoting politicised practice in the health care professions', in E. Rich, L. Monaghan and L. Aphramor (eds) *Debating Obesity: Critical Perspectives*, London: Palgrave Macmillan, 192–218.
Azzarito, L. (2009) 'The rise of the corporate curriculum: fatness, fitness, and whiteness', in J. Wright and V. Harwood (eds) *Biopolitics and the 'Obesity Epidemic'*, London: Routledge, 183–96.
Bakhtin, M. (1965) *Rabelais and His World*, Cambridge, MA: The MIT Press.
Basham, P., Gori, G. and Luik, L. (2006) *Diet Nation: Exposing the Obesity Crusade*, London: The Social Affairs Unit.
Beausoleil, N. (2009) 'An impossible task? Prevented disordered eating in the context of the current obesity panic', in J. Wright and

V. Harwood (eds) *Biopolitics and the 'Obesity Epidemic'*, London: Routledge: 93–107.

Bell, K. and McNaughton, D. (2007) 'Feminism and the invisible fat man', *Body & Society*, 13(1): 107–31.

Bell, K., McNaughton, D. and Salmon, A. (2009) 'Medicine, morality and mothering: public health discourses on foetal alcohol exposure, smoking around children and childhood overnutrition', *Critical Public Health*, 19(2): 155–70.

Boero, N. (2007) 'All the news that's fat to print: the American "obesity epidemic" and the media', *Qualitative Sociology*, 30: 41–60.

—— (2009) 'Fat kids, working moms, and the "epidemic of obesity"', in E. Rothblum and S. Solovay (eds) *The Fat Studies Reader*, New York: New York University Press, 113–19.

Bordo, S. (1993) *Unbearable Weight: Feminism, Western Culture, and the Body*, Berkeley: University of California Press.

Brandon, T. and Pritchard, G. (2011) '"Being fat": a conceptual analysis using three models of disability', *Disability & Society*, 26(1): 79–92.

Brandt, A. and Rozin, P. (eds) (1997a) *Morality and Health*, New York: Routledge.

—— (1997b) 'Introduction', in A. Brandt and P. Rozin (eds) *Morality and Health*, New York: Routledge, 1–11.

Browne, R. (2011) 'Lifting an unfair burden from Generation Next', *The Sun-Herald*, 27 November, 8–9.

Burgard, D. (2009) 'What is "Health at Every Size"?', in E. Rothblum and S. Solovay (eds) *The Fat Studies Reader*, New York: New York University Press, 42–53.

Burgard, D., Dykewomon, E., Rothblum, E. and Thomas, P. (2009) 'Are we ready to throw our weight around? Fat studies and political activism', in E. Rothblum and S. Solovay (eds) *The Fat Studies Reader*, New York: New York University Press, 334–40.

Burrows, L. (2009) 'Pedagogizing families through obesity discourse', in J. Wright and V. Harwood (eds) *Biopolitics and the 'Obesity Epidemic'*, London: Routledge, 127–40.

Butler, J. (1990) *Gender Trouble: Feminism and the Subversion of Identity*, New York: Routledge.

Bynum, C. (1987) *Holy Feast and Holy Fast: The Religious Significance of Food to Medieval Women*, Berkeley: University of California Press.

Cahill, A. (2010) 'Getting to my fighting weight', *Hypatia*, 25(2): 485–92.

Campos, P. (2004) *The Obesity Myth: Why America's Obsession with Weight is Hazardous to Your Health*, New York: Gotham Books.

—— (2011) 'Does fat kill? A critique of the epidemiological evidence', in E. Rich, L. Monaghan and L. Aphramor (eds) *Debating Obesity: Critical Perspectives*, London: Palgrave Macmillan, 36–59.

Campos, P., Saguy, A., Ernsberger, P., Oliver, E. and Gaesser, G. (2006) 'The epidemiology of overweight and obesity: public health crisis or moral panic', *International Journal of Epidemiology*, 35(1): 55–60.

Chan, N. K.-C. and Gillick, A. (2009) 'Fatness as a disability: questions of personal and group identity', *Disability & Society*, 24(2): 231–43.

Chernin, K. (1981) *Womansize: The Tyranny of Slenderness*, London: The Women's Press.

Colls, R. and Evans, B. (2009) 'Introduction: questioning obesity politics', *Antipode*, 41(5): 1011–20.

Cooper, C. (1997) 'Can a fat woman call herself disabled?', *Disability & Society*, 12(1): 31–42.

—— (2007) 'Headless fatties'. Online. Available: http://www.charlottecooper.net/docs/fat/headless_fatties.htm (accessed 15 January 2012).

—— (2009) 'Maybe it should be called Fat American Studies', in E. Rothblum and S. Solovay (eds) *The Fat Studies Reader*, New York: New York University Press, 327–33.

—— (2010) 'Fat Studies: mapping the field', *Sociology Compass*, 4(12): 1020–34.

Deleuze, G. and Guattari, F. (1985) *Anti-Oedipus*, London: Athlone Press.

—— (1988) *A Thousand Plateaus*, London: Athlone Press.

Department of Health (2011) *Healthy Lives, Healthy People: A Call to Action on Obesity in England*, London: Department of Health.

Ernsberger, P. (2009) 'Does social class explain the connection between weight and health?', in E. Rothblum and S. Solovay (eds) *The Fat Studies Reader*, New York: New York University Press, 25–36.

Evans, B. and Colls, R. (2009) 'Measuring fatness, governing bodies: the spatialities of the Body Mass Index (BMI) in anti-obesity politics', *Antipode*, 41(5): 1051–83.

Evans, B., Colls, R. and Horschelmann, K. (2011) '"Change4Life for your kids": embodied collectives and public health pedagogy', *Sport, Education and Society*, 16(3): 323–41.

Evans, J., Rich, R., Davies, B. and Allwood, R. (2008) *Education, Disordered Eating and Obesity Discourse: Fat Fabrications*, London: Routledge.

Farrell, A. (2009) '"The white man's burden": female sexuality, tourist postcards, and the place of the fat woman in early 20th-century U.S. culture', in E. Rothblum and S. Solovay (eds) *The Fat Studies Reader*, New York: New York University Press, 256–62.

Featherstone, M. (2010) 'Body, image and affect in consumer culture', *Body & Society*, 16(1): 193–221.

Foucault, M. (1973) *The Birth of the Clinic: An Archaeology of Medical Perception*, London, Tavistock.

—— (1988) 'Technologies of the self', in L. Martin, H. Gutman and P. Hutton (eds) *Technologies of the Self: A Seminar with Michel Foucault*, London: Tavistock, 145–62.

—— (1991) 'Governmentality', in G. Burchell, C. Gordon and P. Miller (eds) *The Foucault Effect: Studies in Governmentality*, Hemel Hempstead: Harvester Wheatsheaf, 87–104.

Fullagar, S. (2009) 'Governing healthy family lifestyles through discourses of risk and responsibility', in J. Wright and V. Harwood (eds) *Biopolitics and the 'Obesity Epidemic'*, London: Routledge, 108–26.

Gaesser, G. (2002) *Big Fat Lies: The Truth about Your Weight and Your Health*, Carlsbad, CA: Gurze Books.

Gailey, J. (2012) 'Fat shame to fat pride: fat women's sexual and dating experiences', *Fat Studies*, 1(1): 114–27.

Gard, M. (2009) 'Friends, enemies and the cultural politics of critical obesity research', in J. Wright and V. Harwood (eds) *Biopolitics and the 'Obesity Epidemic'*, London: Routledge, 31–44.

—— (2010) 'Truth, belief and the cultural politics of obesity scholarship and public health policy', *Critical Public Health*, 21(1): 37–48.

—— (2011) *The End of the Obesity Epidemic*, London: Routledge.

Gard, M. and Wright, J. (2005) *The Obesity Epidemic: Science, Morality and Ideology*, London: Routledge.

Gill, R. (2008) 'Body talk: negotiating body image and masculinity', in S. Riley, M. Burns, H. Frith, S. Wiggins and P. Markula (eds) *Critical Bodies: Representations, Identities and Practices of Weight and Body Management*, Houndmills: Palgrave Macmillan, 101–16.

Gilman, S. (2010) *Obesity: The Biography*, Oxford: Oxford University Press.

Gimlin, D. (2008) 'Older and younger women's experiences of commercial weight loss', in S. Riley, M. Burns, H. Frith, S. Wiggins and P. Markula (eds) *Critical Bodies: Representations, Identities and Practices of Weight and Body Management*, Houndmills: Palgrave Macmillan, 175–92.

Goffman, E. (1963) *Stigma: Notes on the Management of Spoilt Identity*, London: Penguin.

Grosz, E. (1994) *Volatile Bodies: Toward a Corporeal Feminism*, St Leonards: Allen & Unwin.

—— (1995) *Space, Time & Perversion: The Politics of Bodies*, Sydney: Allen & Unwin.

Guthman, J. (2009a) 'Neoliberalism and the constitution of contemporary bodies', in E. Rothblum and S. Solovay (eds) *The Fat Studies Reader*, New York: New York University Press, 187–96.

—— (2009b) 'Teaching the politics of obesity: insights into neoliberal embodiment and contemporary biopolitics', *Antipode*, 41(5): 1110–33.

Guthman, J. and DuPuis, M. (2006) 'Embodying neoliberalism: economy, culture, and the politics of fat', *Environment and Planning D: Society and Space*, 24: 427–48.

Halse, C. (2009) 'Bio-citizenship: virtue discourses and the birth of the bio-citizen', in J. Wright and V. Harwood (eds) *Biopolitics and the 'Obesity Epidemic'*, London: Routledge, 45–59.

Hartley, C. (2001) 'Letting ourselves go: making room for the fat body in feminist scholarship', in J. Braziel and K. LeBesco (eds) *Bodies Out of Bounds: Fatness and Transgression*, Berkeley: University of California Press, 60–73.

Harwood, V. (2009) 'Theorizing biopedagogies', in J. Wright and V. Harwood (eds) *Biopolitics and the 'Obesity Epidemic'*, London: Routledge, 15–30.

Herrick, C. (2009) 'Shifting blame/selling health: corporate social responsibility in the age of obesity', *Sociology of Health & Illness*, 31(1): 51–65.

Hesse-Biber, S. (1996) *Am I Thin Enough Yet? The Cult of Thinness and the Commercialization of Identity*, New York: Oxford University Press.

Hetrick, A. and Attig, D. (2009) 'Fat bodies, classroom desks, and academic excess', in E. Rothblum and S. Solovay (eds) *The Fat Studies Reader*, New York: New York University Press, 197–204.

Holland, K., Blood, R.W., Thomas, S., Lewis, S., Komesaroff, P. and Castle, D. (2011) '"Our girth is plain to see": an analysis of newspaper coverage of *Australia's Future "Fat Bomb"*, *Health, Risk & Society*, 13(1): 32–46.

Holm, S. (2007) 'Obesity interventions and ethics', *Obesity Reviews*, 8(Suppl. 1): 207–10.

Huang, R.-C., Stanley, F. and Beilin, L. (2009) 'Childhood obesity in Australia remains a widespread health concern that warrants population-wide prevention programs', *Medical Journal of Australia*, 191(1): 45–47.

Huff, J. (2009) 'Access to the sky: airplane seats and fat bodies as contested spaces', in E. Rothblum and S. Solovay (eds) *The Fat Studies Reader*, New York: New York University Press, 176–86.

Inthorn, S. and Boyce, T. (2010) '"It's disgusting how much salt you eat!": television discourses of obesity, health and morality', *International Journal of Cultural Studies*, 13(1): 83–100.

Jallinoja, P., Pajari, P. and Absetz, P. (2010) 'Negotiated pleasures in health-seeking lifestyles of participants of a health promoting intervention', *Health*, 14(2): 115–30.

Johnston, J. and Taylor, J. (2008) 'Feminist consumerism and fat activists: a comparative study of grassroots activism and the Dove Real Beauty campaign', *Signs*, 33(4): 941–66.

Jutel, A. (2006) 'The emergence of overweight as a disease category: measuring up normality', *Social Science and Medicine*, 63: 2268–76.

—— (2009) 'Doctor's orders: diagnosis, medical authority and the exploitation of the fat body', in J. Wright and V. Harwood (eds) *Biopolitics and the 'Obesity Epidemic'*, London: Routledge, 60–77.

Keenan, J. and Stapleton, H. (2010) 'Bonny babies? Motherhood and nurturing in the age of obesity', *Health, Risk & Society*, 12(4): 369–83.

Kent, L. (2001) 'Fighting abjection: representing fat women', in J. Braziel and K. LeBesco (eds) *Bodies Out of Bounds: Fatness and Transgression*, Berkeley: University of California Press, 130–50.

Kirkland, A. (2011) 'The environmental account of obesity: a case for feminist skepticism', *Signs*, 36(2): 463–85.

Klein, R. (2001) 'Fat beauty', in J. Braziel and K. LeBesco (eds) *Bodies Out of Bounds: Fatness and Transgression*, Berkeley: University of California Press, 19–38.

Kristeva, J. (1982) *Powers of Horror: An Essay in Abjection*, New York: Columbia University Press.

Kulick, D. (2005) 'Porn', in D. Kulick and A. Meneley (eds) *Fat: The Anthropology of an Obsession*, New York: Jeremy P. Tarcher/Penguin, 77–92.

Kulick, D. and Meneley, A. (2005) 'Introduction', in D. Kulick and A. Meneley (eds) *Fat: The Anthropology of an Obsession*, New York: Jeremy P. Tarcher/Penguin, 1–8.

Leahy, D. (2009) 'Disgusting pedagogies', in J. Wright and V. Harwood (eds) *Biopolitics and the 'Obesity Epidemic'*, London: Routledge, 172–82.

LeBesco, K. (2001) 'Queering fat bodies/politics', in J. Braziel and K. LeBesco (eds) *Bodies Out of Bounds: Fatness and Transgression*, Berkeley: University of California Press, 74–87.

Longhurst, R. (2001) *Bodies: Exploring Fluid Boundaries*, London: Routledge.

—— (2005) 'Fat bodies: developing geographical research agendas', *Progress in Human Geography*, 29(3): 247–59.

Lupton, D. (1994) *Moral Threats and Dangerous Desires: AIDS in the News Media*, London: Taylor & Francis.

—— (1995) *The Imperative of Health: Public Health and the Regulated Body*, London: Sage.

—— (1996) *Food, the Body and the Self*, London: Sage.

—— (1999) *Risk*, London: Routledge.

—— (2004) '"A grim health future": food risks in the Sydney press', *Health, Risk & Society*, 6(2): 187–200.

—— (2012) *Medicine as Culture: Illness, Disease and the Body*, 3rd edition, London: Sage.

McNaughton, D. (2011) 'From the womb to the tomb: obesity and maternal responsibility', *Critical Public Health*, 21(2): 179–90.

Madden, H. and Chamberlain, K. (2010) 'Nutritional health, subjectivity and resistance: women's accounts of dietary practices', *Health*, 14(3): 292–309.

Mallyon, A., Holmes, M., Coveney, J. and Zadoroznyj, M. (2010) 'I'm not dieting, "I'm doing it for science": masculinities and the experience of dieting', *Health Sociology Review*, 19(3): 330–42.

Merleau-Ponty, M. (1962) *The Phenomenology of Perception*, London: Routledge & Kegan Paul.

—— (1968) *The Visible and the Invisible*, Evanston, IL: Northwestern University Press.

Mitchell, A. (2005) 'Pissed off', in D. Kulick and A. Meneley (eds) *Fat: The Anthropology of an Obsession*, New York: Jeremy P. Tarcher/Penguin, 211–25.

Monaghan, L. (2005a) 'Discussion piece: a critical take on the obesity debate', *Social Theory & Health*, 3: 302–14.

—— (2005b) 'Big Handsome Men, Bears and others: virtual constructions of fat male embodiment', *Body & Society*, 11(2): 81–111.

—— (2007) 'Body mass index, masculinities and moral worth: men's critical understandings of "appropriate" weight-for-height', *Sociology of Health & Illness*, 29(4): 584–609.

Monaghan, L. and Hardey, M. (2011) 'Bodily sensibility: vocabularies of the discredited male body', in E. Rich, L. Monaghan and L. Aphramor (eds) *Debating Obesity: Critical Perspectives*, London: Palgrave Macmillan, 60–89.

Mosher, J. (2001) 'Setting free the bears: refiguring fat men on television', in J. Braziel and K. LeBesco (eds) *Bodies Out of Bounds: Fatness and Transgression*, Berkeley: University of California Press, 166–93.

Murray, S. (2005) 'Doing politics or selling out?: Living the fat body', *Women's Studies*, 34(3–4): 265–77.

—— (2008) *The 'Fat' Female Body*, Houndmills: Palgrave Macmillan.

—— (2009a) 'Marked as "pathological": "fat" bodies as virtual confessors', in J. Wright and V. Harwood (eds) *Biopolitics and the 'Obesity Epidemic'*, London: Routledge, 78–90.

—— (2009b) 'Women under/in control? embodying eating after gastric banding', *Radical Psychology*, 8(1). Online. Available: http://www.radicalpsychology.org/vol8–1/murray.html (accessed 30 November 2011).

O'Hara, L. and Gregg, J. (2012) 'Human rights casualties from the "war on obesity": why focusing on body weight is inconsistent with a human rights approach to health', *Fat Studies*, 1(1): 32–46.

Oliver, J. Eric (2006) *Fat Politics: The Real Story Behind America's Obesity Epidemic*, New York: Oxford University Press.

Orbach, S. (1978) *Fat is a Feminist Issue: The Anti-Diet Guide to Permanent Weight Loss*, London: Arrow Books.

Petersen, A. and Lupton, D. (1996) *The New Public Health: Health and Self in the Age of Risk*, London: Sage.

Probyn, E. (2008) 'Silences beyond the mantra: critiquing feminist fat', *Feminism & Psychology*, 18(3): 401–4.

Puhl, R. and Heuer, C. (2010) 'Obesity stigma: important considerations for public health', *American Journal of Public Health*, 100(6): 1019–28.

Rail, G. (2009) 'Canadian youth's discursive constructions of health in the context of obesity discourse', in J. Wright and V. Harwood (eds) *Biopolitics and the 'Obesity Epidemic'*, London: Routledge, 141–56.

Rich, E. and Evans, J. (2009) 'Performative health in schools: welfare policy, neoliberalism and social regulation?', in J. Wright and V. Harwood (eds) *Biopolitics and the 'Obesity Epidemic'*, London: Routledge, 157–71.

Rich, E., Evans, J. and De Pian, L. (2011) 'Children's bodies, surveillance and the obesity crisis', in E. Rich, L. Monaghan and L. Aphramor (eds) *Debating Obesity: Critical Perspectives*, London: Palgrave Macmillan, 139–63.

Ristovski-Slijepcevic, S., Bell, K., Chapman, G. and Beagan, B. (2010) 'Being "thick" indicates you are eating, you are healthy and you have an attractive body shape: perspectives on fatness and food choice amongst Black and White men and women in Canada', *Health Sociology Review*, 19(3): 317–29.

Ritenbaugh, C. (1982) 'Obesity as a culture-bound syndrome', *Culture, Medicine & Psychiatry*, 6(4): 347–61.

Ross, B. (2005) 'Fat or fiction: weighing the "obesity epidemic"', in M. Gard and J. Wright, *The Obesity Epidemic: Science, Morality and Ideology*, London: Routledge, 86–106.

Rothblum, E. (2012) 'Why a journal on fat studies?', *Fat Studies*, 1(1): 3–5.

Saguy, A. and Almeling, R. (2008) 'Fat in the fire: science, the news media and the "obesity epidemic"', *Sociological Forum*, 23(1): 53–83.

Sedgwick, E. Kosofsky (1990) *The Epistemology of the Closet*, Los Angeles: University of California Press.

Shabot, S. Cohen (2006) 'Grotesque bodies: a response to disembodied cyborgs', *Journal of Gender Studies*, 15(3): 223–35.

Shakespeare, T. (2011) 'Nasty, brutish and short?: the predicament of disability and embodiment', paper presented at Reproducing Normality: Disability, Prenatal Testing and Bioethics workshop, University of Sydney, Sydney, 7 December.

Shapiro, S. (1994) 'Re-membering the body in critical pedagogy', *Education and Society*, 12(1): 61–78.

Shildrick, M. (1997) *Leaky Bodies and Boundaries: Feminism, Postmodernism and (Bio)ethics*, London: Routledge.

Shilling, C. (1993) *The Body and Social Theory*, London: Sage.

Snider, S. (2009) 'Fat girls and size queens: alternative publications and the visualizing of fat and queer eroto-politics in contemporary American culture', in E. Rothblum and S. Solovay (eds) *The Fat Studies Reader*, New York: New York University Press, 223–30.

Solovay, S. and Rothblum, E. (2009) 'Introduction', in E. Rothblum and S. Solovay (eds) *The Fat Studies Reader*, New York: New York University Press, 1–7.

Throsby, K. (2008) 'Happy re-birthday: weight loss surgery and the "new me"', *Body & Society*, 14(1): 117–33.

—— (2012) 'Obesity surgery and the management of excess', *Sociology of Health & Illness*, 34(1): 1–15.

Tischner, I. and Malson, H. (2008) 'Exploring the politics of women's in/visible "large" bodies', *Feminism & Psychology*, 18(2): 260–67.

—— (2011) '"You can't be supersized?": exploring femininities, body size and control within the obesity terrain', in E. Rich, L. Monaghan and L. Aphramor (eds) *Debating Obesity: Critical Perspectives*, London: Palgrave Macmillan, 90–114.

Turner, B. (1991) 'The discourse of diet', in M. Featherstone, M. Hepworth and B. Turner (eds) *The Body: Social Processes and Cultural Theory*, London: Sage, 157–69.

Walkerdine, V. (2009) 'Biopedagogies and beyond', in J. Wright and V. Harwood (eds) *Biopolitics and the 'Obesity Epidemic'*, London: Routledge, 199–207.

Wann, M. (2005) 'Fat & choice: a personal essay', *MP: An Online Feminist Journal*. Online. Available: http://academinist.org/wpcontent/uploads/2005/09/010308Wann_Fat.pdf (accessed 30 November 2011).

—— (2009) 'Foreword: Fat Studies: An invitation to revolution', in E. Rothblum and S. Solovay (eds) *The Fat Studies Reader*, New York: New York University Press, ix–xxv.

Warin, M., Turner, K., Moore, V. and Davies, M. (2008) 'Bodies, mothers and identities: rethinking obesity and the BMI', *Sociology of Health & Illness*, 30(1): 97–111.

Webb, H. (2009) '"I've put on weight 'cos I've bin inactive, 'cos I've 'ad me knee done": moral work in the obesity clinic', *Sociology of Health & Illness*, 31(6): 854–71.

Wegenstein, B. and Ruck, N. (2011) 'Physiognomy, reality television and the cosmetic gaze', *Body & Society*, 17(4): 27–55.

INDEX